Copyright 2020 by Bessie Alvarez -All rights reserved.

No part of this book may be reproduced or transmitted in any form or by any means, electronic or mechanical, including photocopying and recording, or by any information storage and retrieval system, without permission in writing from the publisher. This is a work of fiction. Names, places, characters and incidents are either the product of the author's imagination or are used fictitiously, and any resemblance to any actual persons, living or dead, organizations, events or locales is entirely coincidental. The unauthorized reproduction or distribution of this copyrighted work is illegal .

<u>Disclaimer Notice:</u>

Please note the information contained within this document is for educational and entertainment purposes only. All effort has been executed to present accurate, up to date, reliable, complete information. No warranties of any kind are declared or implied. Readers acknowledge that the author is not engaged in the rendering of legal, financial, medical, or professional advice. The content within this book has been derived from various sources. Please consult a licensed professional before attempting any techniques outlined in this book.

CONTENTS

Introduction

Autoimmune diseases have become an epidemic in America. Currently, over 50 to 75 million Americans are distressed by some sort of autoimmune disorder. Autoimmune disease is the 3rd leading chronic illness in the United States, with cancer and heart disease being the other two. In addition, over $100 billion is spent annually in treatment and research.

While there are various kinds of autoimmune disease and disorders (such as lupus, thyroid, rheumatoid arthritis, type 1-diabetes, etc.) they are linked together regarding their immune response that tricks your body to harm itself. Despite the autoimmune disease, the true dilemma (and answer) lies with the body's immune system. Autoimmune disease arises when your immune system is working overtime to fight infectious organisms or dangerous substances, and it cannot distinguish between the perpetrators and your own body parts. The body's immune system converts antibodies from the defenders to the attackers, falsely attacking your own tissues rather than the perpetrators, causing possibly a broad spectrum of symptoms.

The solution to autoimmune disease is to take control of your life. It all begins with your diet and lifestyle choices! And with that said, allow me to introduce you to the autoimmune diet! This diet is not your typical diet, it's not meant for you to lose weight and not to get healthy. Instead, it was created solely to restore your immune system back to its original state to reduce inflammation. However, those who follow the autoimmune diet can lose weight, improve their gut health, balance blood sugar levels, and help regulate their hormones. On this diet, you will restrict a wide range of foods such as nuts, sugar, grains, legumes, nightshade vegetables, and gluten.

In this book, you will learn everything you need to know about the autoimmune disease and how the autoimmune diet can help reduce inflammation in the body. The Autoimmune Diet Instant Pot Cookbook will teach you how to make some of the most delicious meals on the planet and more. It includes a broad array of recipes and the cooking instructions for preparing those delicious dishes. Nutrition information is also provided for every recipe as well. We have done our very best to include a variety of recipes to please everyone. Here you will find nutrient-dense meals ready to be served for breakfast, lunches, and dinner. These recipes include soups, salads, meats, poultry, seafood, vegan, vegetarian, desserts – just about anything you can think of!

These recipes are simple and delicious and go well with the autoimmune diet. At the end of the book, you will find a 3-week autoimmune diet meal plan, which will cleanse your body to learn more about your body and the foods that trigger you. Use this book daily as it contains tons of incredibly delicious recipes that will satisfy your stomach and help you feel better.

<u>Chapter 1: Why Autoimmune Diet?</u>

Many known autoimmune diseases have no cure, and very limited treatment options, as they are not well understood. But many doctors are beginning to encourage those with autoimmune diseases to make simple lifestyle changes, like diet, which can help boost your body's immune system and several autoimmune diseases. In this chapter, you will learn everything about the autoimmune diet, why you should follow it, and how to stick with it. We will cover the following topics:

Everything About Autoimmune Disease and Problems
What is the Autoimmune Diet?
The Best Benefits of the Autoimmune Diet
Foods Allowed on the Autoimmune Diet
Foods That Should Be Avoided on the Autoimmune Diet
Tips and Tricks to Successfully Follow the Autoimmune Diet
Autoimmune Diet FAQs
Let's begin!

Everything About Autoimmune Disease and Problems

What are autoimmune diseases?
The immune system defends the body from infections and disease. However, those suffering from autoimmune disease, the immune system mistakenly attacks healthy cells in your body which can affect various parts of the body. This is not the usual reaction of the body's immune system, and autoimmune disorders can quickly damage the immune system, and eventually other systems in the body. Autoimmune diseases can have serious consequences both physically and mentally, and can even lead to death.

Most autoimmune disease don't have a cure and very limited treatment options. Many doctors are beginning to recommend simple lifestyle changes and dietary adjustments to help boost their body's immune system, with any luck, a boost of the body's response when the autoimmune disease start to attack.

What is inflammation?
According to Dr. Rhonda Patrick of Found My Fitness, inflammation is the response of your body's immune system to an injury, whether it's from a toxin, infection or tissue damage. Chronic inflammation was believed to be the main cause of pain and discomfort in our joints and muscles. It is also the underlying cause of autoimmune disease, cancer, obesity, heart disease, asthma attacks, Alzheimer's and allergies.

Inflammation can be beneficial as it defends our bodies against viruses and bacteria. It also assists in restoring our bodies. For instance, if you cut yourself, the body sends white blood cells to the site of injury, to kill off any dangerous bacteria from entering your body. This process is known as "acute inflammation," which is essential for how our bodies heal itself.

However, chronic inflammation is a different process. It doesn't protect nor heal our bodies. Rather it attacks our very own cells. Chronic inflammation is where white blood cells attack the body, where blood vessels thicken, developing clogged arteries and scar tissues, lessening the mobility of key organs.

Chronic inflammation is linked to many health problems including joint pain, muscle pain, immune system diseases and disorders. Other issues linked between inflammation and autoimmune issues include rheumatoid arthritis, lupus, celiac disease, leaky gut syndrome, migraines, irritable bowel syndrome, chronic fatigues, and more.

Living with chronic inflammatory or autoimmune conditions is difficult, most of these conditions cause a host of problems. This makes day-t0-day living tough, even for hardy people.

Some symptoms for those suffering from inflammatory issues or autoimmune conditions, include the following:
Joint pain
Muscle pain
Abdominal pain
Weight loss and weight gain
Temperature intolerance (hot or cold)
Skin hives and skin rashes
Hair loss
Mouth ulcers (or canker sores)
Weakness or extreme fatigue
Body tremors, trembling, and shaking
Diarrhea
Frequent urination
Bloody stool

Fast heart rate
Dry mouth, dry eyes, dry skin
Infertility
Lack of focus
Pimples and acne
Dizziness
Blood clots

What is the Autoimmune Diet?

The best way to fight against autoimmune disease is with the autoimmune paleo or AIP diet. This diet sole purpose is to reduce inflammation, which in turn strengthens the immune system among other things. The autoimmune diet can achieve good health, lose weight, increase energy, and reduce or eliminate chronic inflammatory symptoms that may be the leading factor in autoimmune disease. This diet will help restore healthy bacteria to your gut intestines and allow you to learn more about your body.

This diet also focuses on nutrient-rich, unprocessed, and anti-inflammatory foods, such as vegetables. Regardless whether you are suffering from an autoimmune disease or not, you will benefit from following this diet. Beginning this diet, you would try the AIP diet for a couple of weeks to cleanse your body before incorporating foods outside of the AIP diet. This will allow you to learn more about what foods trigger your body more than others.

The autoimmune protocol diet limits grains, legumes, dairy, processed foods, refined sugars, seed oils, nightshade vegetables, nuts and seeds, and eggs. You will be replacing all these foods with nutrient-dense and healthier foods such as vegetables, herbs, coconut products, vinegar, chicken, and beef. Due to the number of restrictions on this diet, it may be tough for you to follow. You might find it troublesome to stick through it, especially when it comes across your everyday living.

The absolute best thing you can do to fight autoimmune disease and disorders is to take care of yourself. Take control of your own life, your own health, and your own future. It all begins with the foods you put in your body.

The Best Benefits of the Autoimmune Diet

The autoimmune diet comes with many health benefits. As the autoimmune diet restricts several food groups and encourages dieters to eat more anti-inflammatory foods and nutrient-dense vegetables they will find physical and mental improvements. For those suffering from an autoimmune disease, this can create a whole new world for them. Here are the different issues that the autoimmune diet tackles:

Restores your immune system: The autoimmune diet will include essential microorganisms to your gut, fix the intestinal barrier and give off the necessary micronutrients that your immune system needs to run properly.

Balances your hormones: The autoimmune diet can help balance your hormones, which in turn, helps the immune system regulate itself. Even better, following the autoimmune diet for the long-term will achieve optimal hormonal balance.

Achieves good health: The autoimmune diet is loaded with nutrient-dense foods and tons of vegetables. The more nutrient-dense foods you eat, the more you provide your body and the body's immune system something to work with. This will help correct body imbalances and nutritional deficiencies that are presently ruining your immune system.

Detoxification: Since your body takes in fewer toxins, your body can effectively eliminate existing toxins.

Balanced blood sugar levels: By getting rid of sugar, your body will start to use healthy fats and protein to provide the body with the energy it needs.

In addition to these benefits, you will boost your metabolism, improve nutrient absorption, improve focus and increase energy, with so much more!

Foods Allowed on the Autoimmune Diet

Below you will learn some of the best foods allowed on the autoimmune diet that can help boost your immune system. Refer to this section whenever you are confused on what you can eat and what you cannot eat while on the autoimmune diet:

Vegetables: Eating a ton of vegetables is a known natural remedy to reverse and prevent autoimmune diseases since they are packed with nutrients and fiber that allow our bodies to thrive. On the Autoimmune Diet, it is recommended to eat nine servings of vegetable per day. Vegetables allowed are:

- Any cruciferous vegetables
- Artichokes
- Asparagus
- Avocados
- Beet
- Broccoli
- Brussel sprouts
- Bok choy
- Cabbage
- Carrots
- Cauliflower
- Swiss chard
- Cucumber
- Fennel
- Kale
- Leek
- Lettuce
- Mushroom
- Pumpkin
- Onion
- Spinach
- Squash
- Sweet potatoes
- Turnips
- Mustard greens
- Watercress
- Avocados
- All kinds of sea vegetables
- Seed form of green beans and peas

Specific Herbs and Spices: You should add as many herbs and spices to your meals. Not only will this enhance the flavor of your food but their tastes are known to support autoimmune conditions and prevent disease. Consider the following herbs and spices:

- Balm (Lemon balm)
- Basil
- Bay leaves
- Chamomile
- Chervil
- Coriander
- Cinnamon
- Cloves
- Dill weed
- Garlic
- Ginger
- Horseradish
- Lavender
- Marjoram leaves
- Onion powder
- Oregano leaves

- Parsley
- Peppermint
- Rosemary
- Saffron
- Sage
- Salt
- Savory leaves
- Spearmint
- Tarragon thyme
- Turmeric

Temporary herbs and spices you can add to your meals are the following:

- Allspice
- Black pepper
- Caraway
- Cardamom
- Green peppercorns
- Juniper
- Pink peppercorns
- Star anise
- Vanilla bean
- White pepper

Protein: Organic and naturally pastured fed proteins contains gut-healing properties. On the Autoimmune Diet, it is recommended for 5 servings of protein per week. Include the following quality meat (organic, pasture-fed, grass-fed) to your diet:

- Poultry
- Beef
- Buffalo
- Chicken
- Duck
- Lamb
- Pheasant
- Pork
- Rabbit
- Turkey
- Wild boar
- Organ meat and offal
- All kinds of wild fish and shellfish (It is recommended for 3 servings of wild fish and shellfish per week)
- Glycine-rich foods including connective tissue, joints, organ meats, etc.

Healthy Fats: Healthy fats are essential for a well-balanced diet. They help reinstate gut wall cells and help absorbs vitamins including vitamin A, vitamin D, vitamin K, and vitamin E! In addition, healthy fats make us feel satiated and satisfied! Here are some good sources of healthy fats:

- Olives
- Olive oils
- Truffle oil
- Coconut oil
- Avocados
- Coconut
- Fatty Fish
- Organic animal fats

Fruit: Fruits are loaded with many important nutrients such as potassium, folate, and vitamin C. However, some studies suggest that you should totally remove fruit from your diet, while other research suggests you should have 2 servings per day. Some good fruits include:

- Apples
- Avocados
- Bananas
- All kinds of berries (Blueberries, blackberries, cranberries, strawberries, etc.)
- Cherries
- Citrus fruits such as lemon, lime, etc.

- Dates
- Coconut
- Fig
- Grapes
- Kiwifruit
- Mangoes
- Melons
- Peaches
- Pears
- Plums
- Pineapples
- Pomegranates
- And watermelon!

Other Foods: Other foods that are allowed on the Autoimmune Protocol Diet are the following:
- Vinegar such as apple cider vinegar, balsamic vinegar, and red wine vinegar
- Arrowroot starch
- Tapioca starch
- Coconut flour
- Coconut sugar
- Coconut palm sugar
- Dried fruits
- Raw honey
- Organic maple syrup

To recap, foods that are highly encouraged on the AIP diet are:
- Organic meats and wild-caught fish
- Vegetables (Excluding nightshade vegetables)
- Sweet potatoes!
- Fruits (Only in few quantities)
- Coconut milk
- Olive oil, avocado oil, and coconut oil (Avoid every other oil)
- Dairy-free fermented foods
- Honey/maple syrup
- Non-seed herbs including basil, oregano, and mint
- Non-seed herbal teas
- Low-sodium bone broth
- Vinegar such as apple cider vinegar

Foods That Should Be Avoided on the Autoimmune Diet

The Autoimmune Diet is an extremely limited diet and can be hard to follow. There is a long list of foods that you should limit and or absolutely avoid! This diet is sort of similar with the paleo diet, such as:

- Gluten
- Grains
- Beans and legumes
- Dairy products
- Processed foods
- Sugars
- Seed Oils

The Autoimmune diet also restricts the following foods, which is not necessarily prohibited in the paleo diet, such as:

- Whole eggs
- Nuts and seeds
- Coffee
- Certain spices
- Nightshade vegetables
- Gums
- Artificial sweeteners and food thickeners

Here's the definitive list of the foods you should keep an eye on during the AIP diet:

Gluten and Grains: Gluten is absolutely prohibited on the autoimmune diet. Research has shown that gluten can trigger an autoimmune disease, damage the liver, and even damage the brain. Avoid the following:

- Wheat
- Wheat germ
- Rye
- Spelt
- Graham
- Barley
- All-purpose flour
- Yeast
- Cornstarch
- Potato starch
- All sorts of pasta (even ravioli, couscous, gnocchi, and dumplings)
- All sorts of noodles (including ramen, udon noodles, soba noodles, rice noodles, egg noodles, and Chow Mein)
- All bread and pastries (even banana bread, potato bread, muffins, flatbreads, bagels, pita, naan, croissants, and donuts)
- All crackers (even pretzels, graham crackers, animal crackers, and goldfish)
- Baked goods (including cakes, cookies, doughnuts, pie crusts, and brownies)
- All cereal and granola (including corn flakes, rice crispy, oats, bran flakes, etc.)
- All sorts of breakfast foods (including pancakes, French toast, waffles, biscuits, and crepes)
- Panko breadcrumbs
- Croutons and stuffing
- Store-bought sauces and gravies
- Store-bought salad dressings and marinades
- Canned soups
- Candy and candy bars
- Potato chips
- French fries
- Energy bars and granola bars
- Traditional soy sauces
- Flour tortillas
- Beer
- Cheesecake filling
- Tortilla chips

- Quinoa

The following are commonly mistaken as high-gluten ingredients, but are allowed in the AIP diet:

- Caramel colors
- Distilled vinegar
- Dextrin
- Maltodextrin
- Natural flavors
- Yeast extract

Nightshade Vegetables: Research suggests that nightshade vegetables can trigger an inflammatory response in the body. Limit or avoid the following nightshade vegetables:

- All kinds of tomatoes
- Bell peppers
- Eggplants
- Goji berries
- Hot peppers such as jalapeno peppers and habanero peppers
- Cape gooseberries
- Tomatillos
- Potatoes
- Paprika seasoning
- Red pepper flakes seasoning
- Paprika seasoning

Herbs and Spices: Some herbs and spices that are not generally allowed on the AIP diet are the following:

- Anise seed
- Annatto seed
- Black caraway seasoning
- Cayenne pepper seasoning
- Celery seeds
- Chili pepper flakes
- Chili powder
- Ground coriander
- Coriander seeds
- Curry powder
- Ground cumin
- Cumin seeds
- Dill seed
- Fennel seed
- Fenugreek
- Mustard seed
- Nutmeg
- Paprika
- Poppy seed
- Sesame seed

Dairy: On the AIP diet, you will eliminate dairy due to the linked it has with autoimmune diseases, inflammatory responses in the body, and arthritis. You will avoid the following:

- Whole dairy milk
- Butter
- Margarine
- Cream
- Cottage cheese
- Condensed milk
- Half and half
- Heavy cream
- Milk powder
- Nonfat milk
- Yogurt
- Whey
- Sour cream

- All kinds of cheeses such as cheddar cheese, Monterey Jack cheese, mozzarella cheese, blue cheese, etc.)

The closest thing you can have to dairy is ghee (non-clarified butter)!

Legumes: People with autoimmune diseases should avoid legumes due to their high inflammatory content. Avoid the following:

- Most legumes are restricted on the autoimmune diet, however peas and green beans still in seed form are allowed.
- Asparagus beans
- Asparagus peas
- Baby lima beans
- Black beans
- Black-eyed peas
- Boston beans
- Broad beans
- Cannellini beans
- Chickpeas
- Chili beans
- Cranberry beans
- Fava beans
- Kidney beans
- Lentils
- Lima beans
- Mexican black beans
- Mung beans
- Navy beans
- Pinto beans
- Red kidney beans
- Scarlet runner beans
- Snow peas
- Soybeans
- White kidney bean
- Peanuts
- Chickpeas

Nuts and Seeds: Some doctors suggest that you restrict your intake of nuts and seeds due to their anti-nutrient content, this includes:

- Brazil nuts
- Pine nuts
- Chestnuts
- Macadamia nuts
- Pistachios
- Almonds
- Pecans
- Walnut
- Cashew
- Acorns
- Sesame
- Sunflower seeds
- Pumpkin seeds

This also means limit or restrict nuts and seeds products such as:

- Nut milk (Almond milk, cashew milk, etc.)
- Nut and seed oils (Almond oil, avocado oil, canola oil, corn oil, cottonseed oil, grapeseed oil, etc.)
- Nut and seed flours such as almond flour
- Nut butter
- Cocoa

Sugar: It's no surprise that sugar should be avoided. Sugar is not good for autoimmune conditions. You should avoid the following sugars:

- White sugar
- Brown sugar
- Powdered sugar

- Barley sugar
- Caramel
- High-fructose syrup
- Molasses
- Organic Turbinado sugar
- Agave nectar

If you absolutely need to sweeten a beverage you can use honey, maple syrup, or coconut palm sugar.

Artificial Sweeteners: While artificial sweeteners are not as worse as refined sugar, you should still limit your intake of artificial sweeteners. This includes:

- Stevia sweetener
- Erythritol sweetener
- Xylitol sweetener
- Splenda sweetener

Other foods to limit or avoid on the AIP Diet are the following:

- Alcohol
- White eggs
- Thickeners and emulsifiers
- Food additives
- Rice
- Coffee (Instant coffee, espresso, etc.)
- Oats
- Potatoes
- Quinoa
- Rice
- Tapioca
- Vegetable oil

Tips and Tricks to Successfully Follow the Autoimmune Diet

Embarking on the autoimmune diet can be daunting. It's also very hard to successfully stick with it due to their number of food restrictions. Here you will learn some of the top tips and tricks for surviving the autoimmune diet:

Meal plan: It is highly recommended that you plan your meals days and sometimes weeks ahead. Figure out what you want to eat at what time of the day and be sure there are tons of vegetables and anti-inflammatory meals on the menu.

Treat yourself. This cookbook contains fun and easy AIP-friendly dessert recipes for you to enjoy! Allow yourself to relax each week by eating something you really want to enjoy.

Sleep: Research shows that it will be to your benefit to sleeping for 7 to 8 hours per night. To get the most out of your sleep, make sure you set an alarm to wake you up in the morning and prepare your bed beforehand. Research has also found that reading a book rather than checking your Instagram feed late at night will make you go to sleep faster.

It's a great idea to store prepared meals in your freezer for whenever you are hungry or being tempted to eat something you don't want to. For example, if you are making soup for dinner. Store the leftovers in a mason jar and heat it for your next meal.

Stress Management: Studies have found that stress can be a trigger of autoimmune disease. It is critical that you keep your stress levels low to maintain good health. I recommend for everyone to begin meditating and practice yoga. Try becoming more mindful of your daily activities, both emotionally and physically.

Keep a food journal. In this food journal, you will write what you eat, your feelings while eating, how you feel immediately after consuming it, how you felt 1 to 3 hours after eating, and how you adjusted to dietary changes and cravings on the autoimmune diet.

Autoimmune Diet FAQs

How long do I have to follow the autoimmune diet?
The autoimmune diet was created as an elimination diet to learn about your body's food intolerances. It is recommended to restrict foods for 30 days and then reintroduce items back to your diet one at a time to figure out whether they have any negative reactions.

What's the difference between the paleo diet and the autoimmune diet?
While both diets are incredibly similar, the autoimmune protocol diet is an elimination diet. The goal is to reduce inflammation and to learn what is causing inflammatory reactions.

The Paleo Diet
The AIP diet follows the Paleo Diet guidelines with the addition of:

- Nuts and seeds
- Eggs
- Nightshade vegetables
- Caffeine

I have constipation due to the AIP diet. How can I deal with this?
Constipation is a common side effect due to a huge dietary change. Here are some ways to deal with it:

- Ensure you're consuming enough vegetables and fruits
- Drink plenty of water
- Ensure you're consuming enough healthy fats
- Drink prune juice

Can I eat out while on the AIP diet?
It is recommended to avoid eating out at restaurants as restaurant dishes contains nondisclosed ingredients. If you must dine out, tell the water that you are on a strict diet. Ask for your meals to be prepared using olive oil or coconut oil rather than vegetable oil. Politely ask them not to add specific seasonings such as paprika, cayenne pepper, black pepper, etc.

Can I add black pepper to my meals?
Adding black pepper to your meals is completely up to you. You may find some of the recipes in this cookbook asking for you to add them in. But do take note that some people have noted that black pepper was the leading cause of inflammation. Always be cautious of what you put in your body.

If I cheat on the AIP diet, do I have to restart?
Yes, unfortunately. Elimination diets are very strict on the rules and you must avoid the foods for at least 30 consecutive days. This is the only way to accurately learn about your food intolerances.

Chapter 2: Why Instant Pot?

The Instant Pot is a truly sensational kitchen appliance. It can cook many foods in a sealed chamber in only a matter of minutes. In this chapter, you will learn everything about the Instant Pot, why you should use it, and how to use it. We will cover these following topics:

Everything About the Instant Pot and How it Works

Benefits of Using an Instant Pot

What Does Each Instant Pot Button Do?

The Best Instant Pot Tips and Tricks

The Definitive Instant Pot Cooking Timetable

If you are already a professional Instant Pot user, you can go ahead and skip this chapter. With that said, let's begin!

Everything About the Instant Pot and How It Works

Literally, everyone is talking about the extraordinary Instant Pot! The Instant Pot is an all-in-one kitchen appliance that performs the capabilities of many different kitchen appliances which includes:

- Pressure Cookers
- Rice Cookers
- Slow Cookers
- Sauté/Browning Pans
- Yogurt Makers
- Steamers
- Warmers

You can literally put your crockpot and rice cookers in storage once you acquire the Instant Pot!This 7-in-1 Multi-Functional Pressure Cooker promises to cook foods up to 70 percent faster with fewer energy. It was designed with safety and easy cooking in mind It can also release hot steam in ease – which truly is something too dangerous to perform on a traditional stove-top pressure cooker.

Not only does the Instant Pot prepare dishes up to 70 percent quicker to support a hectic lifestyle. The Instant Pot makes foods by utilizing hot steam in an airtight environment which enriches the flavor of food, makes it healthier and cooks food quicker.

The Instant Pot comes with 14 Smart Programs, which includes:

- Soup/Broth Button
- Meat/Stew Button
- Bean/Chili Button
- Poultry Button
- Sauté/Simmer Button
- Rice Button
- Multigrain Button
- Porridge Button
- Steam Button
- Slow Cook Button
- Keep Warm Button
- Yogurt Button
- Manual Button
- And Pressure Cook Button

Now your favorite meals can be completed with the single push of a button!

Why Should You Own an Instant Pot?

The Instant Pot is a truly remarkable kitchen appliance that comes with numerous benefits. Explore the many benefits of cooking your meals with an Instant Pot.

- **Speed:** The Instant Pot promises that it cooks foods up to 70 percent faster when using the pressure cooking setting. How the Instant Pot achieves this speedy cooking is that it builds up pressure inside an airtight chamber which surrounds food in a high temperature which results in fast cooking.
- **Versatility:** The Instant Pot is a 7-in-1 Multi-functional pressure cooker which has the capabilities of the following: slow cookers, rice cookers, yogurt maker, sauté/browning, steamer, warmer, and pressure cooker.
- **Less Energy:** The Instant Pot uses less energy which can save you money on your electric bill.
- **Healthier Meals:** Foods are trapped in a sealed container which means nutrients, vitamins and minerals are preserved resulting in healthier foods.
- **Safer Foods:** Pressure cooking can help kill off any harmful microorganisms and bacteria lurking in glass containers and food.

What Does Each Instant Pot Button Do?

Is the Instant Pot something new to your kitchen? Or perhaps you are familiar with the Instant Pot, but don't know what all those buttons do? In this section, if you're ever confused on the buttons in the future. Here you will learn what every Instant Pot Button do.

Button	Function
Sauté	The Sauté button is used to sauté vegetables, brown meat, and simmer ingredients in the Instant Pot without the lid. You can use the "Adjust" button to set to one of these three temperatures: "normal", "more", and "less".
Manual	The Manual button is used to pressure cook foods at High Pressure. Most of the recipes in this cookbook will ask for you to press this button.
Keep Warm/Cancel	This button is used to cancel any function or turn off the Instant Pot.
[-] and [+]	This button is used to adjust the cooking time.
Less | Normal | More	This button is used to adjust the cooking temperature by repeatedly selecting the button until the desired cooking temperature is reached.
Soup/Broth	This button will cook for 30 minutes at High Pressure.
Meat/Stew	This button will cook for 35 minutes at High Pressure.
Bean/Chili	This button will cook for 30 minutes at High Pressure.
Poultry	This button will cook for 15 minutes at High Pressure.
Rice	This function is used to cook rice at Low Pressure using your Instant Pot. The cooking time will depend on water volume and rice inside your Instant Pot.
Multigrain	This button will cook for 30 minutes at High Pressure
Porridge/Congee	This button will cook for 20 minutes at High Pressure.
Steam	This function is used to cook for 10 minutes at High Pressure. Use this button with a steamer rack or trivet inside your Instant Pot.
Slow Cook	This function is used to slow cook your meals and is automatically set for 4 hours.
Yogurt	This button is selected for yogurt making. Read your Instant Pot manual to learn how to use this function.
Cake	This button cook food for 40 minutes at High Pressure. (Only found in newer Instant Pot models)
Egg	This button cooks for 4 minutes at High Pressure. (Only found in newer Instant Pot models)
Sterilize	This button is used to sterilize cooking utensils and pasteurized milk for yogurt making. (Only found in newer Instant Pot models)
Pressure/Pressure Level Button:	This button is used to adjust between High Pressure and Low Pressure.
Timer Button/Delay Start	This button can be used to set the timer on your Instant Pot and delay cooking for up to 24 hours.

How to Cook Using Your Instant Pot?

The Instant Pot is incredibly easy to use. Here's the common procedure you need to take to pressure cook foods inside your Instant Pot.
1.   Add the desired foods to your Instant Pot.
2.   Close and seal the lid.
3.   Press the desired setting and cooking time.
4.   Press start and allow the Instant Pot electric pressure cooker to cook your foods. It will take 10 to 40 minutes for your Instant Pot to reach the pressure level before the official cooking starts.
5.   When your Instant Pot beeps, it's done. Release the pressure (read below) and carefully remove the lid.
6.   Voila!

There are two methods for releasing pressure from your Instant Pot. As pressure builds up inside your electric pressure cooker it will need de-pressurize before you remove the lid. The two methods include:
•   **Quick-Release:** To quick-release the pressure, all you need to do is switch the valve from "sealing" to "venting." This procedure only takes a minute or so.
•   **Natural Release:** The natural release method is where the Instant Pot depressurizes gradually over time. This procedure takes around 10 to 30 minutes depending on the liquid volume in the inner pot. The more liquid content, the longer it takes to release all the pressure. Some recipes in this cookbook require you to natural release the pressure before you quick release the remaining pressure. This allows the food inside your Instant Pot to cook a bit longer in the sealed environment.

Some other pointers when using your Instant Pot:

Functions: The Instant Pot kitchen appliance can perform many functions including slow cooking, sautéing/browning, pressure cooking, warming foods, steaming foods, making yogurt, rice making, sterilizer, cake making, and egg cooking

Programs: The Instant Pot comes with numerous distinctive programs. Different cooking programs that can save you time in the kitchen. For example, if you are preparing a soup all you need to do is press the "Soup/Broth" button.

Control Panel: The control panel allows you to navigate and control the cooking process. It allows you to change the settings of your Instant Pot and contains information regarding pressure levels, operation keys, function keys, and mode.

Best Instant Pot Tips and Tricks

If you're lucky enough to own an Instant Pot electric pressure cooker, you know how useful these kitchen appliances are. The Instant Pot can replace multiple kitchen appliances, saving you space in your kitchen and money. Here you will learn some of the most useful tips and tricks for using your Instant Pot.
•   Don't overfill your Instant Pot. Be attentive to the maximum level marking in your Instant Pot. The inner pot should never be over 2/3 full whenever you are pressure cooking.
•   Always make sure at least ½ cup of liquid (water, broth, soup, wine, etc.) is inside the inner pot before pressure cooking. Pressure is created by steam gradually building up in the airtight chamber.
•   Be familiar with your Instant Pot functions. This will save you a whole lot of time and energy in the long run rather than reading the manual repeatedly.
•   Plan before you use your Instant Pot. Make sure you fully read each recipe before you begin to cook. Some recipes might call for some supplies or ingredients you don't necessarily have at the moment.
•   It's not necessary to defrost your foods before using pressure cooking in your Instant Pot. However, you do need to add a couple more minutes to the cooking time.
•   It takes around 10 to 40 minutes for your Instant Pot to build up the pressure, so make sure you consider the pressure building time, the cooking time, and pressure releasing time when you are making meals.
•   When using the sauté setting, make sure the inner pot is greased with olive oil, butter, or ghee before sautéing the vegetables or searing the meat.
•   Many recipes ask for you to sauté onions/garlic/aromatics/vegetables. Sauté these vegetables using the Instant Pot on the low sauté mode.
•   To enhance the flavor of your meats, use the sauté function to brown your meats first before you begin the pressure cooking process.
•   To reduce sauces and liquids using your Instant Pot, press the sauté button and allow to cook until you reach the desired consistency, stirring occasionally.
•   It can take a lengthy amount of time for your Instant Pot to build up the pressure. You can speed up the pressure building process by pressing the sauté function to heat your ingredients. Once at the desired

temperature, press the "Keep Warm/Cancel" button, close the lid, press the manual button, and select the cooking time.
- Make sure you take care of your Instant Pot. You can wash the inner pot, steam rack, and other Instant Pot accessories in your dishwasher. To get rid of the funky smell of the unit, you can use white vinegar, boiling water, or lemon.
- Ensure the pressure valve is switched to the "sealing" position. If you are pressure cooking and it's not on the "sealing" position, your Instant Pot won't be able to build up pressure properly.
- Never open your Instant Pot during the cooking process. If you remove the lid during the cooking process, hot steam will hit your face. Make sure the pressure is either quickly or naturally released before removing the lid.
- Learn the difference between quick release pressure method and natural release pressure method. Only use the natural pressure release when cooking soups, stews, or foods with large liquid volume.

The Definitive Instant Pot Cooking Timetable

The Instant Pot is a truly amazing kitchen appliance. It cooks foods twice as fast with an even more deliciousness added to the mouth. When using frozen foods with your Instant Pot, you don't necessarily need to defrost using a microwave. It's as simple as dumping the ingredients in the multicooker and pressing a few buttons. To make a proper and delicious meal, it is essential to plan appropriately.

Please note that the cooking time can vary based on the following factors:
- Various cuts of meat (Chuck, flank, ribs, brisket, etc.)
- Various kinds of rice (Brown rice, Arborio rice, basmati (white) rice, whole grain rice, etc.)
- Various kinds of legumes (Beans, chickpeas, kidney beans, etc.)
- Amounts of liquid inside the Instant Pot chamber
- Natural pressure release or quick pressure release

Taste preferences differ from individual to individual. People want to taste different things and want different texture and tenderness of foods. Your Instant Pot can surely help you achieve this. The cooking timetable you find below is meant for cooking reference only. I highly encourage all Instant Pot users to play around with their multicookers and figure out the best cooking procedures for their own preferred foods.

Below you will find the pressure-cooking time for the following groups of food:
- Dry beans, legume, and lentils
- Meat (Poultry, Pork, Beef, and Lamb)
- Fish and Seafood
- Grains and Rice
- Vegetables (Fresh or Frozen)
- Fruits (Fresh or Frozen)

Fish and Seafood	Cooking Time for Fresh Ingredients (in minutes)	Cooking Time for Frozen Ingredients (in minutes)
Whole crab	2 to 3 minutes	4 to 5 minutes
Whole fish	4 to 5 minutes	5 to 7 minutes
Fish fillet	2 to 3 minutes	3 to 4 minutes
Fish steak	3 to 4 minutes	4 to 6 minutes
Lobster	3 to 4 minutes	4 to 6 minutes
Mussels	2 to 3 minutes	Not available
Shrimp/Prawns	1 to 3 minutes	2 to 4 minutes
Low-Sodium Seafood Stock	7 to 8 minutes	8 to 9 minutes

Grains and Rice	Water Quantity Ratio (Grain: Water)	Cooking Time for Grains and Rice (in minutes)
Pearly barley	1: 2.5	20 to 22 minutes
Pot barley	1:3 to 1:4	25 to 30 minutes
Thick congee	1:4 to 1:5	15 to 20 minutes
Thin congee	1:6 to 1:7	15 to 20 minutes
Couscous	1:2	2 to 3 minutes
Dried corn or halved corn	1:3	5 to 6 minutes
Whole Kamut	1:2	10 to 12 minutes
Millet	1: 1.75	10 to 12 minutes

Quick-cooking oats	1: 1.5	2 to 3 minutes
Steel-cut oats	2: 2.5	3 to 5 minutes
Thin porridge	1:2	10 to 15 minutes
Quick-cooking quinoa	1: 1.25	1 minute
Basmati rice	1:1	4 minutes
Brown rice	1:1	22 to 25 minutes
Jasmine rice	1:1	4 minutes
White rice	1:1	4 minutes
Wild rice	1:1	20 to 25 minutes
Sorghum	1:3	20 to 25 minutes
Unsoaked spelt berries	1: 1.5	25 to 30 minutes
Unsoaked wheat berries	1:3	20 to 25 minutes

Dry Beans, Legume, and Lentils	Cooking Time for Dry Ingredients (in minutes)	Cooking Time for Soaked Ingredients (in minutes)
Adzuki beans	16 to 20 minutes	4 to 6 minutes
Anasazi beans	20 to 25 minutes	5 to 7 minutes
Black beans	20 to 25 minutes	6 to 8 minutes
Black-eyed peas	10 to 15 minutes	4 to 5 minutes
Chickpeas	35 to 40 minutes	10 to 15 minutes
Cannellini beans	30 to 35 minutes	8 to 10 minutes
Great northern beans	25 to 30 minutes	8 to 10 minutes
Red kidney beans	25 to 30 minutes	8 to 10 minutes
White kidney beans	30 to 35 minutes	8 to 10 minutes
Cannellini kidney beans	30 to 35 minutes	8 to 10 minutes
Green lentils	10 to 12 minutes	Not available
Brown lentils	1o to 12 minutes	Not available
Split red lentils	5 to 6 minutes	Not available
Split yellow lentils	18 to 12 minutes	Not available
Lima beans	12 to 14 minutes	8 to 10 minutes
Navy beans	20 to 25 minutes	7 to 8 minutes
Pinto beans	25 to 30 minutes	8 to 10 minutes
Peas	6 to 10 minutes	Not available
Scarlet runner	20 to 25 minutes	8 to 10 minutes
Soybeans	35 to 46 minutes	18 to 20 minutes

Meat (Poultry, Pork, Beef, and Lamb)	Cooking Time (in minutes)
Stew meat beef	20 minutes
Beef meatballs	8 to 10 minutes
Dressed beef	20 minutes
Beef (pot roast, steak, round, brisket), cut into small chunks	15 minutes
Beef (pot roast, steak, round, brisket), cut into large chunks	20 minutes
Rib beef	20 to 25 minutes
Beef Shanks	25 to 30 minutes
Beef, oxtail	40 to 50 minutes
Boneless chicken breast	8 minutes
Chickens, cut with bones	10 to 15 minutes
Chicken stock	40 to 45 minutes
Duck, cut with bones	12 to 15 minutes
Duck, whole	10 minutes
Ham, sliced	9 to 12 minutes
Ham, picnic shoulder	8 minutes
Lamb, stew meat	12 to 15 minutes

Lamb's Leg	15 minutes
Pheasant	8 minutes
Pork loin roast	20 minutes
Pork butt roast	15 minutes
Pork ribs	15 to 20 minutes
Boneless turkey breast	7 to 9 minutes
Whole turkey breast	20 to 25 minutes
Turkey legs or drumsticks	15 to 20 minutes
Veal Chops	5 to 8 minutes
Veal roast	12 minutes
Whole quail	8 minutes

Vegetables	Fresh Cooking Times (in minutes)	Frozen Cooking Times (in minutes)
Whole, trimmed artichokes	9 to 11 minutes	11 to 13 minutes
Artichoke hearts	4 to 5 minutes	5 to 6 minutes
Whole or cut asparagus	1 to 2 minutes	2 to 3 minutes
Whole, trimmed green beans	1 to 2 minutes	2 to 3 minutes
Small whole beetroot	11 to 13 minutes	13 to 15 minutes
Large whole beetroot	20 to 25 minutes	25 to 30 minutes
Broccoli florets	1 to 2 minutes	2 to 3 minutes
Broccoli stalks	3 to 4 minutes	4 to 5 minutes
Whole brussel sprouts	2 to 3 minutes	3 to 4 minutes
Shredded green, red, or purple cabbage	2 to 3 minutes	3 to 4 minutes
Wedged green, red, or purple cabbage	3 to 4 minutes	4 to 5 minutes
Sliced or shredded carrots	2 to 3 minutes	3 to 4 minutes
Whole or chunked carrots	6 to 8 minutes	7 to 9 minutes
Cauliflower florets	2 to 3 minutes	3 to 4 minutes
Celery chunks	2 to 3 minutes	3 to 4 minutes
Collard greens	4 to 5 minutes	5 to 6 minutes
Corn kernels	1 to 2 minutes	2 to 3 minutes
Corn on the cob	3 to 5 minutes	4 to 6 minutes
Sliced or chunked eggplants	3 to 4 minutes	3 to 4 minutes
Endive	1 to 2 minutes	2 to 3 minutes
Chopped escarole	2 to 3 minutes	3 to 4 minutes
Whole green beans	2 to 3 minutes	3 to 4 beans
Chopped greens	2 to 3 minutes	4 to 7 minutes
Leeks	2 to 3 minutes	3 to 4 minutes
Mixed vegetables	3 to 4 minutes	4 to 6 minutes
Okra	2 to 3 minutes	3 to 4 minutes
Sliced onions	2 to 3 minutes	3 to 4 minutes
Chunked parsnips	3 to 4 minutes	4 to 5 minutes
Peas in the pod	1 to 2 minutes	2 to 3 minutes
Green peas	1 to 2 minutes	2 to 3 minutes
Cubed potatoes	3 to 4 minutes	4 to 5 minutes
Whole baby potatoes	8 to 10 minutes	12 to 14 minutes
Whole large potatoes	12 to 15 minutes	15 to 19 minutes

Fruits	Fresh Cooking Time (in minutes)	Dried Cooking Time (in minutes)
Apple slices or chunks	1 to 2 minutes	2 to 3 minutes
Whole apples	3 to 4 minutes	4 to 6 minutes
Whole apricot	2 to 3 minutes	3 to 4 minutes
Peaches	2 to 3 minutes	4 to 5 minutes
Whole pears	3 to 4 minutes	4 to 6 minutes

Pear slices or halves	2 to 3 minutes	4 to 5 minutes
Plums	2 to 3 minutes	4 to 5 minutes
Raisins	Not available	4 to 5 minutes

Chapter 3: Delicious Autoimmune Diet Recipes

Breakfast Recipes

Morning Sweet Potato Breakfast Bowls

Time: 20 minutes
Servings: 4
Ingredients:
4 medium sweet potatoes, cleaned
1 cup of water
A small pinch of sea salt
1/2 teaspoon of organic ground cinnamon powder
2 tablespoons of maple syrup or pure organic honey
Banana slices (Topping)
Instructions:
1.	Place a wire rack insert or a steamer basket in your Instant Pot pressure cooker.
2.	Place the sweet potatoes on top and pour in the 1 cup of water.
3.	Cover and seal the lid on your Instant Pot.
4.	Press the "Manual" button and cook for 15 minutes on High Pressure.
5.	When the cooking is done, wait for 5 minutes before quick-releasing the pressure and removing the lid.
6.	Carefully remove the sweet potatoes.
7.	Scoop the sweet potato flesh away from the skin and place to a bowl.
8.	Add the salt, cinnamon powder, and honey. Mash until reached your desired consistency.
9.	Top with banana slices.
10.	Serve and enjoy!
Nutrition information per serving:
- Calories: 293
- Fat: 0.5g
- Carbohydrates: 69.3g
- Protein: 9.6g
- Dietary Fiber: 3.4g

Optimum Chicken and Apple Meatballs

Time: 20 minutes
Servings: 4
Ingredients:
1-1/2 pound of ground chicken
3 tablespoons of coconut oil
1 medium apple, peeled, cored and finely chopped
2 tablespoons of dried oregano
2 tablespoons of dried thyme
2 tablespoons of dried parsley
1 teaspoon of garlic powder
1/2 teaspoon of sea salt
1/2 teaspoon of freshly cracked black pepper
1/4 cup of homemade low-sodium chicken broth or water
Instructions:
1. Press the "Sauté" function on your Instant Pot and add 1 tablespoon of coconut oil.
2. Add the finely chopped apples to the Instant Pot along with the dried herbs. Sauté for 6 to 8 minutes or until softened, stirring occasionally.
3. Remove the apples from the Instant Pot and turn off.
4. In a large bowl, combine the chicken with the apples, garlic powder, salt, and black pepper.
5. Form the mixture into meatballs.
6. Press the "Sauté" function on your Instant Pot and add the remaining 2 tablespoons of coconut oil.
7. Working in batches, if necessary, add the meatballs and cook until no longer pink.
8. Add the chicken broth.
9. Close and seal the lid. Press the "Manual" button and cook for 5 minutes at High Pressure.
10. When the timer beeps, quick release or naturally release the pressure and remove the lid.
11. Serve and enjoy!
Nutrition information per serving:
- Calories: 412
- Fat: 30g
- Carbohydrates: 15g
- Protein: 26g
- Dietary Fiber: 2g

Gratifying Kale Butternut Squash and Pancetta Breakfast Hash

Time: 30 minutes

Servings: 6

Ingredients:

1 pound of butternut squash, peeled, deseeded, and cubed

1 large bunch of fresh kale, roughly chopped

2 garlic cloves, minced

1/2 medium onion, finely chopped

4 medium bacon slices, thickly sliced

1 tablespoon of olive oil or coconut oil

1/4 cup of water or low-sodium vegetable broth

2 teaspoons of apple cider vinegar

1 teaspoon of sea salt

1 teaspoon of freshly cracked black pepper

Instructions:

1.   Press the "Sauté" function on your Instant Pot and add the oil.

2.   Once hot and ready, add the bacon and cook until brown and crispy, stirring occasionally. Remove and set aside

3.   Add the butternut squash cubes, onion, and garlic to your Instant Pot. Sauté until lightly tender, stirring occasionally.

4.   Stir in the roughly chopped kale, vegetable broth, and apple cider vinegar to your Instant Pot.

5.   Allow to cook until the liquid is reduced, the squash is tender, and the kale has wilted, typically around 5 minutes.

6.   Stir in the bacon, sea salt, and freshly cracked black pepper.

7.   Serve and enjoy!

Nutrition information per serving:

- Calories: 169
- Fat: 7.7g
- Carbohydrates: 14.6g
- Protein: 6.9g
- Dietary Fiber: 2.4g

Palatable Maple Bacon Banana Breakfast Muffins

Time: 30 minutes

Servings: 6

Ingredients:

3 large ripe bananas, mashed

2-1/2 cups of coconut flour

1 teaspoon of baking soda

1/4 cup of pure maple syrup or raw honey

6 medium bacon slices, cooked and finely chopped

1/2 cup of unsweetened coconut yogurt

1/2 cup of unsweetened coconut milk

A small pinch of sea salt

Instructions:

1.   Grease individual muffin cups or ramekins with nonstick cooking spray.

2.   In a large bowl, add the mashed bananas, coconut flour, baking soda, maple syrup, bacon slices, coconut yogurt, coconut milk, and sea salt.

3.   Gently stir until fully combined.

4.   Divide and pour the batter into the muffin cups or ramekins.

5.   Add 1 cup of water and a trivet to your Instant Pot.

6.   Place the muffin cups or ramekins on top of the trivet.

7.   Cover and seal the lid. Cook at High Pressure for 25 minutes.

8.   When the cooking is done, naturally release the pressure for 10 minutes before quick releasing the remaining pressure.

9.   Remove the muffins and allow to cool.

10.   Serve and enjoy!

Nutrition information per serving:

- Calories: 396
- Fat: 16.9g
- Carbohydrates: 50.3g
- Protein: 18g
- Dietary Fiber: 13.5g

Highly Regarded Cauliflower and Sweet Potato Breakfast Hash

Time: 20 minutes
Servings: 6

Ingredients:

6 large sweet potatoes
2 tablespoons of coconut oil or olive oil
1 large cauliflower head, cut into florets
1 large onion, finely chopped
6 medium bacon slices, finely diced
3 garlic cloves, minced
1/2 cup of homemade low-sodium vegetable stock
2 teaspoons of freshly squeezed lemon juice
3 tablespoons of fresh rosemary
3 tablespoons of fresh basil
1 teaspoon of sea salt
1 teaspoon of freshly cracked black pepper

Instructions:

1. Press the "Sauté" function on your Instant Pot and add the oil.
2. Once the oil is hot and ready, add the garlic and onions. Sauté until softened, stirring occasionally.
3. Add the sweet potatoes and cauliflower to the Instant Pot.
4. Add the bacon to the Instant Pot along with the salt, black pepper, rosemary, and basil. Sauté for a few minutes, stirring occasionally.
5. Add the vegetable stock and lemon juice to the Instant Pot.
6. Cover and cook on High Pressure for 10 minutes.
7. When the cooking is done, quick release or naturally release the pressure. Remove the lid.
8. Drain the liquid and transfer the vegetables to a serving bowl.
9. Serve and enjoy!

Nutrition information per serving:

- Calories: 353
- Fat: 12.9g
- Carbohydrates: 49.5g
- Protein: 12.1g
- Dietary Fiber: 9.7g

<u>Smoothies, Juices, and Other Beverages Recipes</u>

Delicious Blueberry Coconut Smoothie

Time: 5 minutes
Servings: 1
Ingredients:
1 cup of unsweetened coconut milk
1 cup of frozen blueberries
2 cups of raw spinach or kale
2 tablespoons of coconut butter
1/2 of a large frozen banana
A dash of organic ground cinnamon powder
Instructions:
1.   In a blender, add the coconut milk, frozen blueberries, spinach, coconut butter, banana, and cinnamon powder.
2.   Blend until smooth.
3.   Serve and enjoy!
Nutrition information per serving:
- Calories: 942
- Fat: 85.3g
- Carbohydrates: 50g
- Protein: 11.5g
- Dietary Fiber: 9g

Healthy Green Detox Smoothie

Time: 5 minutes
Servings: 1
Ingredients:
1 medium apple, cored, seeded, and chopped
1 medium cucumber, peeled and cubed
1/2 medium lime, freshly squeezed
1/2 medium lemon, freshly squeezed
1 tablespoon of fresh ginger, minced
1 cup of kale, roughly chopped
1 cup of coconut water
Instructions:
- In a blender, add all chopped apples, cubed cucumbers, lime juice, lemon juice, ginger, kale, and coconut water.
- Blend until smooth.
- Serve and enjoy!
Nutrition information per serving:
- Calories: 270
- Fat: 1.6g
- Carbohydrates: 63.1g
- Protein: 7.1g
- Dietary Fiber: 12.3g

Everyday Avocado Coconut Smoothie

Time: 5 minutes
Servings: 1
Ingredients:
1 medium ripe avocado, peeled and cubed
1 cup of unsweetened coconut milk or unsweetened coconut cream
1/2 cup of coconut water
1 large handful of spinach, lettuce, chard, or kale
4 sprigs of fresh parsley, stemmed
Ice (optional)
Instructions:
1.   In a blender, add the cubed avocado, coconut milk, coconut water, greens, parsley, and ice.
2.   Blend until smooth or reached your desired consistency. Serve and enjoy!
Nutrition information per serving:
- Calories: 963
- Fat: 96.3g
- Carbohydrates: 32.8g
- Protein: 20.1g
- Dietary Fiber: 11g

Perfectly Spiced Apple Cider

Time: 30 minutes
Servings: 6 cups
Ingredients:
6 medium apples, cored and quartered
3 cups of water
1 medium-sized orange, juice and zest
1/4 cup of pure raw honey or maple syrup
1 inch fresh ginger, thinly sliced
2 whole cinnamon sticks
6 whole cloves
A tiny pinch of salt
Instructions:
1.   Add the quartered apple and water to a blender.
2.   Blend until smooth and completely combined.
3.   Strain the contents using a fine mesh strainer into a large pot. Repeat this process three times.
4.   Add the strained apple juice to your Instant Pot along with the orange juice, orange zest, raw honey, ginger, whole cinnamon sticks, cloves, and salt.
5.   Select the "Sauté" function and bring to a boil.
6.   Once you see the liquid begin to boil, turn off your Instant Pot.
7.   Cover and seal the lid. Press the "Manual" button and cook for 10 minutes at High Pressure.
8.   When the cooking is done, naturally release the pressure for 15 minutes and then quick release the remaining pressure.
9.   Remove the lid.
10.   Strain the contents of your Instant Pot using a fine mesh strainer into a pitcher.
11.   Pour into a glass or mug. Serve!
Nutrition information per serving:
- Calories: 173
- Fat: 0.4g
- Carbohydrates: 46g
- Protein: 6.3g
- Dietary Fiber: 0.9g

Energizing Apple Carrot Banana Smoothie

Time: 5 minutes
Servings: 1
Ingredients:
1 medium apple, chopped
1/2 medium fresh carrot, cut into bite-sized pieces or ½ cup of baby carrots
1 large ripe banana
1/2 cup of unsweetened coconut milk or unsweetened coconut cream
1/2 tablespoon of coconut butter or coconut oil
A dash of organic ground cinnamon powder
1 cup of ice (optional)
Instructions:
1.   In a blender or food processor, add the apples, carrot, bananas, coconut milk, coconut butter, cinnamon powder, and ice.
2.   Blend until smooth or reached your desired consistency.
3.   Transfer into a glass. Serve and enjoy!
Nutrition information per serving:
- Calories: 584
- Fat: 36.4g
- Carbohydrates: 61.7g
- Protein: 12.3g
- Dietary Fiber: 5.1g

Sunrise Pineapple Smoothie

Time: 5 minutes
Servings: 1
Ingredients:
Juice of 1 medium grapefruit
2 celery stalks with leaves
2 cups of lettuce, spinach, kale, or chard
1 cup of frozen pineapple
1 cup of coconut water
2 teaspoons of pure raw honey
A small pinch of salt
Instructions:
1.   In a blender, add the grapefruit juice, celery, greens, frozen pineapple, coconut water, honey, and salt.
2.   Blend until smooth or until reached your desired consistency.
3.   Serve and enjoy!
Nutrition information per serving:
- Calories: 232
- Fat: 1.1g
- Carbohydrates: 56.2g
- Protein: 7.4g
- Dietary Fiber: 4.2g

Evening Homemade Ginger Ale

Time: 40 minutes
Servings: 4 cups
Ingredients:
1 pound of fresh ginger, unpeeled and finely chopped
2 medium fresh lemons, juiced and peels reserved
2 tablespoons of pure raw honey
4 cups of water
Instructions:
1.   In a food processor, add the lemon juice and chopped ginger.
2.   Process until minced.
3.   Transfer the pureed contents to your Instant Pot along with the pure raw honey and water.
4.   Cover and seal the lid. Press the "Manual" button and cook for 30 minutes at High Pressure.
5.   When the cooking is done, naturally release the pressure and remove the lid.
6.   Strain and transfer the ginger ale to a glass. Serve and enjoy!
Nutrition information per serving:
- Calories: 55
- Fat: 2g
- Carbohydrates: 13g
- Protein: 0.3g
- Dietary Fiber: 0.1g

Refreshing! Agua De Jamaica "Hibiscus Tea"

Time: 20 minutes
Servings: 8
Ingredients:
1 cup of dried hibiscus flowers
8 cups of water
1 cup of coconut palm sugar
1 teaspoon of fresh ginger, finely minced
1 stick of cinnamon
1 medium lime, juice
Ice (to serve)
Instructions:
1.   Add the dried hibiscus flowers, 8 cups of water, coconut palm sugar, finely minced ginger, and cinnamon stick to your Instant Pot.
2.   Cover and seal the lid. Cook at High Pressure for 5 minutes.
3.   When the cooking is done, naturally release the pressure for 10 minutes and then quick release the remaining pressure.
4.   Remove the lid.
5.   Strain the liquid into a glass pitcher and allow to cool.
6.   Squeeze the 1 medium lime and cool with ice cubes.
7.   Serve and enjoy!
Nutrition information per serving:
- Calories: 15
- Fat: 0.35g
- Carbohydrates: 2.32g
- Protein: 0g
- Dietary Fiber: 0g

Homemade Low-Sodium Chicken Broth

Time: 45 minutes
Servings: 1 batch
Ingredients:
1 whole chicken carcass
2 tablespoons of olive oil or coconut oil
1 cup of fresh celery, sliced
1 cup of orange carrots, sliced
1/2 cup of yellow onions, finely chopped
4 whole garlic cloves, minced
1 tablespoon of dried parsley
1 teaspoon of dried marjoram
1 teaspoon of dried rosemary
1 teaspoon of dried thyme
Water
Instructions:
1.   Press the "Sauté" function on your Instant Pot and add the oil.
2.   Once the oil is hot and ready, add the sliced celery, sliced carrots, chopped onions, and minced garlic. Sauté for 2 minutes.
3.   Turn off the "Sauté" function and gently stir in the chicken carcass and herbs.
4.   Fill your Instant Pot 2/3 of the way full with water.
5.   Cover and seal the lid. Press the "Manual" button and cook for 30 minutes at High Pressure.
6.   When the cooking is done, allow for a full natural release method. Remove the lid.
7.   Season the salt with salt and black pepper. You can skip if you prefer.
8.   In a colander over a large bowl or cooking pot, pour the entire Instant Pot contents through the strainer.
9.   Store in containers.
10.   Serve and enjoy!
Nutrition information per serving:
- Calories: 135
- Fat: 15g
- Carbohydrates: 1g
- Protein: 1g
- Dietary Fiber: 0g

Tasty Mushroom Broth

Time: 30 minutes
Servings: 8 cups
Ingredients:
2 pounds of medium white button mushrooms, quartered
8 fresh sprigs of parsley
6 fresh sprigs of thyme
1 bay leaf
6 medium garlic cloves, minced
2 tablespoons of olive oil or coconut oil
1 medium yellow onion, finely chopped
1 medium leek, sliced
1 medium carrot, finely chopped
8 cups of water
1 teaspoon of sea salt
1/2 teaspoon of freshly cracked black pepper
Instructions:
1.	Press the "Sauté" function on your Instant Pot and add the oil.
2.	Once hot and ready, add the onion, leek, carrot, and minced garlic. Sauté until softened, stirring occasionally.
3.	Gently stir in the mushrooms, fresh parsley, fresh thyme, and bay leaf. Sauté for around 4 minutes, stirring occasionally.
4.	Add the water to your Instant Pot.
5.	Cover and seal the lid. Press the "Manual" button and cook for 10 minutes at High Pressure.
6.	When the cooking is done, quick release the pressure and carefully remove the lid.
7.	Season with sea salt and freshly cracked black pepper. Gently stir.
8.	Using a fine-mesh strainer, strain the liquid over a large container or cooking pot
9.	Serve and enjoy!
Nutrition information per serving:
- Calories: 13
- Fat: 0g
- Carbohydrates: 0.9g
- Protein: 0g
- Dietary Fiber: 0.1g

Soup Recipes

Five-Star Onion Soup

Time: 23 minutes
Servings: 8
Ingredients:
2 tablespoons of coconut oil or olive oil
8 cups of yellow onions, sliced
1 tablespoon of balsamic vinegar
6 cups of homemade low-sodium chicken broth or vegetable broth
2 tablespoons of bay leaves
2 sprigs of thyme
1 teaspoon of sea salt
Instructions:
1.   Press the "Sauté" function on your Instant Pot and add the oil and onions. Sauté until translucent, stirring occasionally. Turn off "Sauté" function.
2.   Add the 1 tablespoon of balsamic vinegar to your Instant Pot along with the chicken broth, bay leaves, thyme, and sea salt.
3.   Cover and seal the lid. Select the "Manual" function and cook for 10 minutes at High Pressure.
4.   When the cooking is done, allow for a full natural release. Carefully remove the lid.
5.   Discard the thyme and bay leaves.
6.   Use an immersion blender to puree the soup until smooth.
7.   Serve and enjoy!
Nutrition information per serving:
- Calories: 106
- Fat: 4.6g
- Carbohydrates: 11.4g
- Protein: 4.9g
- Dietary Fiber: 2.5g

Superb Beet and Fennel Soup

Time: 20 minutes
Servings: 6
Ingredients:
2 pounds of beets, peeled and cut into 1-inch chunks
2 tablespoon of olive oil or coconut oil
1 large onion, finely chopped
4 cups of homemade low-sodium vegetable broth
1 large fennel bulb, thinly sliced
1 tablespoon of fresh ginger, minced
1 medium-sized apple, peeled and chopped
1 tablespoon of red wine vinegar
Freshly squeezed juice from ½ lemon
1/2 teaspoon of sea salt
1/2 teaspoon of freshly cracked black pepper
Instructions:
1.   Select the "Sauté" function on your Instant Pot and add the olive oil and fennel. Sauté until softened.
2.   Add the minced garlic and minced ginger to your Instant Pot. Sauté for an additional minute, stirring occasionally.
3.   Add the rest of the ingredients to your Instant Pot and give a good stir.
4.   Cover and seal the lid. Press the "Sauté" function on your Instant Pot and cook for 15 minutes at High Pressure.
5.   When the cooking is done, naturally release the pressure and remove the lid.
6.   Use an immersion blender to puree the soup until smooth.
7.   Serve and enjoy!
Nutrition information per serving:
- Calories: 145
- Fat: 5.1g
- Carbohydrates: 24.6g
- Protein: 5.5g
- Dietary Fiber: 3.3g

Insanely Delicious Sweet Potato Soup

Time: 31 minutes
Servings: 6
Ingredients:
2 pounds of sweet potatoes, peeled and cubed
2 cups of homemade low-sodium chicken broth
4 garlic cloves, minced
2 tablespoons of coconut oil
1 medium-sized onion, finely chopped
1 teaspoon of sea salt
1 teaspoon of freshly cracked black pepper
Instructions:
1. Press the "Sauté" function on your Instant Pot and add the coconut oil and onions. Sauté until translucent, stirring occasionally.
2. Add the garlic and sauté for an additional minute.
3. Add the sweet potatoes, chicken broth, salt, and black pepper to your Instant Pot.
4. Cover and seal the lid. Press the "Manual" button and cook for 15 minutes at High Pressure.
5. When the cooking is done, naturally release the pressure for 10 minutes before quick-releasing the pressure. Carefully remove the lid.
6. Use an immersion blender to puree the soup until smooth.
7. Serve and enjoy!
Nutrition information per serving:
- Calories: 241
- Fat: 5.3g
- Carbohydrates: 44.8g
- Protein: 6.6g
- Dietary Fiber: 4.3g

Heavenly Cream of Chicken and Vegetable Soup

Time: 40 minutes
Servings: 6
Ingredients:
1/2 to 1 pound of boneless skinless chicken breasts
3 tablespoons of olive oil
1 small head of cauliflower, chopped (around 4 cups)
6 cups of homemade low-sodium chicken broth or vegetable broth
2 medium carrots
1 medium zucchini
1 cup of mushrooms
1 medium-sized onion, finely chopped
1 cup of frozen spinach
1 cup of fresh parsley, finely chopped
1 teaspoon of sea salt
1 teaspoon of freshly cracked black pepper
Instructions:
1.   Press the "Sauté" function on your Instant Pot and add the olive oil and chicken. Cook until brown on both sides. Remove and set aside.
2.   Add the remaining tablespoon of olive oil to your Instant Pot. Add the onion, carrots, zucchini, and mushrooms to your Instant Pot. Cook until softened, stirring occasionally
3.   Add the remaining ingredients to your Instant Pot including the cooked chicken.
4.   Cover and seal the lid. Press the "Manual" button and cook at High Pressure for 15 minutes.
5.   When the cooking is done, naturally release the pressure and remove the lid.
6.   Transfer the chicken to a cutting board and shred using two forks.
7.   Use an immersion blender to puree the vegetables until smooth or a little bit of thick.
8.   Stir in the shredded chicken to the soup and adjust the seasoning as needed.
9.   Serve and enjoy!
Nutrition information per serving:
- Calories: 219
- Fat: 9.6g
- Carbohydrates: 9.5g
- Protein: 3.5g
- Dietary Fiber: 24.8g

Exquisite Cabbage Soup with Pork

Time: 30 minutes
Servings: 8
Ingredients:
1 pound of ground pork
2 pounds of sauerkraut, rinsed
4 cups of homemade low-sodium chicken broth
1 large green cabbage head, cored and shredded
2 tablespoons of olive oil or coconut oil
1 medium-sized yellow or sweet onion, finely chopped
2 garlic cloves, minced
1 tablespoon of fresh ginger, peeled and finely minced
1 teaspoon of dried thyme
1 teaspoon of dried oregano
1 teaspoon of sea salt
1 teaspoon of freshly cracked black pepper
Instructions:
1.   Press the "Sauté" function on your Instant Pot and add the olive oil.
2.   Once the oil is hot and ready, add the ground pork. Cook until brown, breaking it apart with a wooden spoon.
3.   Add the minced garlic, onions, and minced ginger to your Instant Pot. Sauté for 5 minutes or until softened, stirring occasionally.
4.   Turn off the "Sauté" function.
5.   Gently combine the sauerkraut, cabbage, chicken broth, dried thyme, dried oregano, sea salt, and black pepper to your Instant Pot.
6.   Close and seal the lid. Press the "Manual" button and cook for 20 minutes at High Pressure.
7.   When the cooking is done, allow for a full natural release and remove the lid.
8.   Gently stir everything together.
9.   Serve and enjoy!
Nutrition information per serving:
- Calories: 173
- Fat: 8g
- Carbohydrates: 8.32g
- Protein: 3g
- Dietary Fiber: 15g

Yummy Apple Ginger Butternut Squash Soup

Time: 35 minutes
Servings: 8
Ingredients:
2 pounds of butternut squash, peeled, seeded, and cubed
2 medium apples, chopped
2 medium-sized carrots, cut into 1-inch pieces
2 tablespoons of fresh ginger, finely minced
1 medium-sized onion, finely chopped
1 tablespoon of coconut oil or olive oil
2 garlic cloves, minced
4 cups of homemade low-sodium vegetable broth
1 teaspoon of sea salt
1/2 teaspoon of freshly cracked black pepper
Instructions:
1.   Press the "Sauté" function on your Instant Pot and add the olive oil and onions. Sauté until soft, typically 4 to 6 minutes.
2.   Add the minced garlic and minced ginger to your Instant Pot. Sauté for an additional minute.
3.   Add the rest of the ingredients to your Instant Pot.
4.   Cover and seal the lid. Select the "Manual" button and cook for 9 minutes at High Pressure.
5.   When the cooking is done, naturally release the pressure for 10 minutes and quick release the remaining pressure. Carefully remove the lid.
6.   Use an immersion blender to puree the soup until smooth.
7.   Serve and enjoy!
Nutrition information per serving:
- Calories: 117
- Fat: 3g
- Carbohydrates: 25g
- Protein: 3g
- Dietary Fiber: 1g

Beautiful Carrot Soup with Lemongrass

Time: 20 minutes
Servings: 4
Ingredients:
1 medium onion, finely chopped
1 2-inch piece lemongrass stick, pounded
1-1/2 pounds of carrots, chopped
1 large sweet potato, cubed
1 celery stalk, chopped
2 garlic cloves, minced
2 cups of homemade low-sodium vegetable broth
1 cup of unsweetened coconut milk
Freshly squeezed juice of a 1/2medium lime
1 teaspoon of sea salt
1 teaspoon of freshly cracked black pepper
Instructions:
1.   Add all the ingredients besides the freshly squeezed lime juice to your Instant Pot. Give a gently stir.
2.   Cover and seal the lid. Select the "Manual" button and cook for 7 minutes at High Pressure.
3.   When the cooking is done, naturally release the pressure for 10 minutes before using the quick pressure release method.
4.   Use an immersion blender to puree the soup until smooth.
5.   Gently stir in the freshly squeezed lime juice and adjust the seasoning as needed.
6.   Serve and enjoy!
Nutrition information per serving:
- Calories: 257
- Fat: 14.6g
- Carbohydrates: 28.8g
- Protein: 3.7g
- Dietary Fiber: 7.2g

The Most Delicious Cauliflower, Bacon and Leek Soup

Time: 30 minutes
Servings: 4
Ingredients:
2 pounds of cauliflower, cut into florets
1/2 pound of bacon, finely chopped
3 leeks, sliced
1 medium-sized yellow onion, finely chopped
4 garlic cloves
4 cups of homemade low-sodium chicken broth or vegetable broth
1 teaspoon of sea salt
1 teaspoon of freshly cracked black pepper
Instructions:
1. Press the "Sauté" function on your Instant Pot.
2. Once hot and ready, add the bacon and cook until brown and crispy.
3. Once the bacon is done, transfer to a plate lined with paper towels to drain the grease.
4. Add the leeks, onions, and garlic to your Instant Pot. Cook until softened, stirring occasionally.
5. Pour in the broth along with cauliflower, sea salt, and black pepper.
6. Cover and seal the lid. Press the "Manual" button and cook for 15 minutes at High Pressure.
7. When the cooking is done, wait for 5 minutes before performing a quick release method. Remove the lid.
8. Use an immersion blender to blend the contents until smooth and creamy.
9. Gently stir in the crumbled bacon.
10. Serve and enjoy!

Nutrition information per serving:
- Calories: 409
- Fat: 24.1g
- Carbohydrates: 23.3g
- Protein: 6.9g
- Dietary Fiber: 26.7g

Paramount Apple Ginger Carrot Sweet Potato Soup

Time: 30 minutes
Servings: 4
Ingredients:
3 medium-sized sweet potatoes, cubed
1 large carrot, peeled and cut into 1-inch pieces
2 apples, peeled, cored, and chopped
2 to 4 tablespoons of fresh ginger, minced
4 cups of homemade low-sodium chicken broth
1 teaspoon of sea salt
1 teaspoon of freshly cracked black pepper
Instructions:
1. Add all the ingredients to your Instant Pot and gently stir until fully combined.
2. Cover and seal the lid. Press the "Manual" button and cook at High Pressure for 15 minutes.
3. When the cooking is done, wait for 5 minutes before quick releasing the remaining pressure.
4. Use an immersion blender to puree the soup until smooth.
5. Season with sea salt and black pepper.
6. Serve and enjoy!

Nutrition information per serving:
- Calories: 217
- Fat: 0.9g
- Carbohydrates: 52.1g
- Protein: 8.4g
- Dietary Fiber: 2.7g

Extraordinary Zucchini Soup

Time: 25 minutes
Servings: 8
Ingredients:
1.   2-1/2 pounds of zucchini, peeled and chopped
2.   1 medium-sized yellow or sweet onion, finely chopped
3.   2 tablespoons of olive oil or coconut oil
4.   4 garlic cloves, minced
5.   4 cups of homemade low-sodium chicken broth or vegetable broth
6.   1/3 cup of fresh basil
7.   1 teaspoon of sea salt
8.   1 teaspoon of freshly cracked black pepper
Instructions:
1.   Press the "Sauté" function on your Instant Pot and add the olive oil.
2.   Once the oil is hot and ready, add the onions and zucchini. Sauté until the onions are translucent, stirring occasionally.
3.   Add the minced garlic and cook for an additional minute.
4.   Gently stir in the chicken broth to your Instant Pot.
5.   Cover and seal the lid. Press the "Manual" button and cook for 8 minutes at High Pressure.
6.   When the cooking is done, wait for 5 minutes before quick releasing the remaining pressure. Carefully remove the lid.
7.   Gently stir in the fresh basil, salt, and black pepper.
8.   Use an immersion blender to puree the soup until smooth.
9.   Serve and enjoy!
Nutrition information per serving:
- Calories: 80
- Fat: 4.6g
- Carbohydrates: 7g
- Protein: 1.9g
- Dietary Fiber: 4.4g

Salad Recipes

Enjoyable Kale and Pork Salad

Time: 1 hour and 30 minutes
Servings: 6
Pork Ingredients:
4 pounds of boneless pork shoulder, cut into 3 large pieces
1 tablespoon of garlic powder
Fresh zest of 1 medium-sized lime
1 tablespoon of freshly squeezed lime juice
2 tablespoons of olive oil or coconut oil
3/4 cup of unsweetened coconut milk
3 tablespoons of fish sauce
2 teaspoons of sea salt
Salad Ingredients:
1 large bunch of kale, stemmed and roughly chopped
1/2 medium-sized red cabbage, shredded
2 medium-sized zucchini, thinly sliced
Dressing Ingredients:
1/3 cup of unsweetened coconut milk
2 tablespoons of freshly squeezed lime juice
1/3 cup of avocado oil
A small pinch of sea salt
2 teaspoons of fish sauce
Instructions:
1.	Season the pork shoulder with garlic powder, lime zest, and salt.
2.	Press the "Sauté" function on your Instant Pot and add the olive oil.
3.	Once the oil is hot and ready, add the pork to your Instant Pot and cook until brown.
4.	Add the lime juice, fish sauce, and unsweetened coconut milk to your Instant Pot.
5.	Cover and seal the lid. Press the "Manual" button and cook for 90 minutes at High Pressure.
6.	When the cooking is done, quick release the pressure and remove the lid. Remove the pork from the liquid. You can store the liquid in your refrigerator for future use.
7.	Transfer the pork to a cutting board and shred into large chunks or smaller pieces.
8.	To make the dressing: In a bowl, add and combine the coconut milk, lime juice, avocado oil, sea salt, and fish sauce.
9.	In a large bowl, combine the kale, shredded red cabbage, thinly sliced zucchini, pork pieces, and dressing.
10.	Serve and enjoy!
Nutrition information per serving:
- Calories: 71
- Fat: 34.8g
- Carbohydrates: 14.1g
- Protein: 4.3g
- Dietary Fiber: 83g

Comforting Coleslaw Salad with Pulled Chicken

Time: 20 minutes
Servings: 6
Ingredients:
2 tablespoons of coconut oil or avocado oil
1 pound of boneless, skinless chicken breasts
1/4 cup of homemade low-sodium chicken broth
1/2 large green cabbage head, cored and finely shredded
1/2 large red cabbage head, cored and finely shredded
1 large carrot, grated
1 cup of unsweetened coconut milk or unsweetened coconut cream
1/4 cup of apple cider vinegar
2 tablespoons of raw honey
1/2 teaspoon of sea salt
Instructions:
1.   Season the chicken with salt.
2.   Press the "Sauté" function on your Instant Pot and add the coconut oil.
3.   Once the oil is hot, add the chicken breast and cook until brown on both sides.
4.   Add ¼ cup of chicken broth.
5.   Lock the lid and ensure the valve is sealed. Press the "Manual" button and cook at High Pressure for 10 minutes.
6.   When the cooking is done, naturally release the pressure for 5 minutes before quick releasing the rest of the pressure.
7.   Transfer the chicken to a cutting board and shred using two forks. Set aside to a serving platter.
8.   In a large bowl, add the shredded green cabbage, red cabbage, grated carrot, coconut milk, apple cider vinegar, and sea salt. Stir until combined.
9.   Serve the pulled chicken with the coleslaw.
10.   Serve and enjoy!
Nutrition information per serving:
- Calories: 276
- Fat: 16.5g
- Carbohydrates: 9.4g
- Protein: 24.3g
- Dietary Fiber: 3.4g

Captivating Steamed Broccoli Salad with Apple

Time: 20 minutes
Servings: 6
Ingredients:
4 cups of broccoli or 1 large broccoli head, washed and cut into florets
1 cup of water
1 teaspoon of sea salt
3 medium-sized apples, finely chopped
1/4 cup of red onions, finely chopped
1/2 cup of dried cranberries
Dressing Ingredients:
1/4 cup of apple cider vinegar
1/2 cup of coconut oil or olive oil
2 garlic cloves, minced
1 tablespoon of raw honey or pure maple syrup
1/2 teaspoon of sea salt
Instructions:
1.   Add 1 cup of water and a steamer basket to your Instant Pot.
2.   Place the broccoli florets in the steamer basket and sprinkle with sea salt.
3.   Lock the lid and ensure the valve is closed. Press the "Manual" button and adjust the time to 0 minutes at High Pressure. Press start.
4.   Meanwhile, in a small bowl, add all the dressing ingredients and mix until fully incorporated.
5.   When your Instant Pot beeps, quick release the pressure and remove the lid.
6.   In a large bowl, add the steamed broccoli, apples, red onions, and dried cranberries.
7.   Drizzle the dressing.
8.   Serve and enjoy!
Nutrition information per serving:
- Calories: 344
- Fat: 25g
- Carbohydrates: 32g
- Protein: 5.9g
- Dietary Fiber: 6.32g

Thoughtful Sweet Potato Salad

Time: 20 minutes
Servings: 10
Ingredients:
1-1/2 cups of water
5 pounds of sweet potatoes, peeled and cubed
1 pound of cucumbers, chopped
1 cup of homemade AIP mayonnaise
1/2 cup of red onions, finely chopped
1/2 teaspoon of sea salt
1/2 teaspoon of freshly cracked black
Instructions:
1.   Add 1-1/2 cups of water and a steamer basket to your Instant Pot.
2.   Place the sweet potatoes on top of the steamer basket and sprinkle with salt and black pepper.
3.   Cover and seal the lid. Press the "Manual" button and cook for 4 minutes at Highs Pressure.
4.   When the cooking is done, quick release the pressure and remove the lid.
5.   Transfer the sweet potato cubes to a large bowl and allow to cool
6.   Add the remaining ingredients and gently stir until fully combined.
7.   Cover and chill inside your refrigerator until cool.
8.   Serve and enjoy!
Nutrition information per serving:
- Calories: 366
- Fat: 8.3g
- Carbohydrates: 70.53g
- Protein: 9.6g
- Dietary Fiber: 4g

Fascinating Beet Salad with Arugula

Time: 35 minutes
Servings: 6
Beet Ingredients:
6 medium-sized beets, trimmed
Dressing Ingredients:
3 tablespoons of balsamic vinegar
4 tablespoons of olive oil
1 garlic clove, minced
1/4 teaspoon of sea salt
1/4 teaspoon of freshly cracked black pepper
1/4 teaspoon of pure raw honey or maple syrup
Salad Ingredients:
6 cups of arugula
Instructions:
1.   In a bowl, add the balsamic vinegar, olive oil, minced garlic, salt, black pepper, and honey. Stir until fully combined and set aside.
2.   Add 1 cup of water and a steamer basket to your Instant Pot.
3.   Place the beets on your steamer basket.
4.   Close and seal the lid. Press the "Manual" button and cook for 15 minutes at High Pressure.
5.   When the cooking is done, quick release the pressure and remove the lid.
6.   Remove the beets and allow the beets to cool.
7.   Once the beets are cool, remove the skin and cut into 1/2-inch pieces
8.   In a large bowl, combine the arugula and beets.
9.   Drizzle the dressing. Serve and enjoy!
Nutrition information per serving:
- Calories: 314
- Fat: 28g
- Carbohydrates: 16g
- Protein: 7.32g
- Dietary Fiber: 5g

Fun and Easy Kale Steak Salad with Peaches

Time: 20 minutes
Servings: 2
Ingredients:
3 large handfuls of kale, stemmed and roughly chopped
2 medium peaches, chopped
1 beef flank steak, cut in half
1 tablespoon of olive oil or coconut oil
1/2 teaspoon of sea salt
1/2 teaspoon of freshly cracked black pepper.
Salad dressing, olive oil, or balsamic vinegar for dressing
Instructions:
1.   Season the beef flank steak with salt and black pepper.
2.   Press the "Sauté" function on your Instant Pot and add the olive oil and steak. Cook on both sides for 2 to 3 minutes or until brown. Remove and set aside.
3.   Add the peaches to your Instant Pot and sauté for a few minutes. Remove and set aside. Turn off your Instant Pot.
4.   In a large bowl, add the cooked peach, cooked steak, kale, and dressing of choice. Gently stir until fully combined. Serve and enjoy!
Nutrition information per serving:
- Calories: 264
- Fat: 10.1g
- Carbohydrates: 28g
- Protein: 18.3g
- Dietary Fiber: 4.3g

Gentle Shrimp Salad with Fennel, Mango, and Avocado

Time: 8 minutes
Servings: 4
Ingredients:
1 pound of shrimp, peeled and deveined
3 tablespoons of freshly squeezed lime juice
1/2 cup of fresh cilantro, finely chopped
2 tablespoons of fish sauce
1/2 large fennel bulb, thinly sliced
1 medium-sized mango, peeled and cubed
1/2 cup of red onion, thinly sliced
1 large ripe avocado, peeled and cubed
1/4 cup of low-sodium sea stock, chicken broth, or plain ordinary water.
Instructions:
1.   Ade the shrimp and cooking liquid of choice to your Instant Pot.
2.   Lock the lid and ensure the valve is closed. Press the "Manual" button and cook at High Pressure for 5 minutes.
3.   When the cooking is done, quick release the pressure and carefully remove the lid.
4.   Transfer the shrimp to a large bowl and discard the liquid.
5.   Add the lime juice, cilantro, fish sauce, thinly sliced fennel, cubed mango, sliced red onion, and cubed avocado to the bowl. Gently stir until fully combined. Serve and enjoy!
Nutrition information per serving:
- Calories: 231
- Fat: 4g
- Carbohydrates: 21.3g
- Protein: 26.3g
- Dietary Fiber: 2.3g

Highly Recommended Garlic Shrimp Zoodle Salad

Time: 10 minutes
Servings: 4
Ingredients:
1 pound of large shrimp, peeled and deveined
1 tablespoon of freshly squeezed lemon juice
2 tablespoons of coconut oil
4 garlic cloves, minced
2 to 3 medium-sized zucchinis, spiralized
1/2 teaspoon of fresh or dried basil
1/2 teaspoon of fresh or dried oregano
Instructions:
1.	Press the "Sauté" function on your Instant Pot and add 1 tablespoon of coconut oil.
2.	Once the oil is hot and ready, add the garlic and sauté until fragrant, stirring occasionally. Turn off the "Sauté" function and add the shrimp.
3.	Lock the lid and ensure the valve is sealed. Press the "Manual" button and cook at High Pressure for 4 minutes.
4.	When the cooking is done, naturally release the pressure and carefully remove the lid.
5.	Transfer the shrimp to a large bowl.
6.	Press the "Sauté" function on your Instant Pot and add the remaining tablespoon of coconut oil.
7.	Add the spiralized zucchini and sauté until softened. Transfer to a large bowl and top with shrimp. Sprinkle dried basil and dried oregano.
8.	Serve and enjoy!
Nutrition information per serving:
- Calories: 222
- Fat: 9g
- Carbohydrates: 7.7g
- Protein: 27.8g
- Dietary Fiber: 1.7g

Determined Carrot Salad with Dried Cranberries and Pineapples

Time: 10 minutes
Servings: 6
Ingredients:
2 pounds of carrots, peeled and thinly sliced
2 to 4 tablespoons of olive oil
2 garlic cloves, minced
1 tablespoon of apple cider vinegar
1/2 cup of dried cranberries
1/3 cup of fresh pineapples, finely chopped
1/2 cup of AIP-friendly mayonnaise
2 cups of arugula
Instructions:
1.	Press the "Sauté" function on your Instant Pot and add the olive oil, garlic, apple cider vinegar, and carrots. Sauté for 6 to 8 minutes or until tender, stirring occasionally.
2.	Turn off your "Sauté" setting on your Instant Pot and transfer the carrots to a large bowl.
3.	Add the dried cranberries, chopped pineapples, mayonnaise, and arugula. Gently stir until fully combined.
4.	Serve and enjoy!
Nutrition information per serving:
- Calories: 121
- Fat: 6.9g
- Carbohydrates: 26.32g
- Protein: 4.63g
- Dietary Fiber: 2.3g

Unique Taco Salad

Time: 20 minutes
Servings: 6
Ingredients:
1 pound of extra-lean ground beef
1 romaine lettuce head, chopped
1 medium-sized avocado, cubed
1/4 cup of onions, finely chopped
1-1/2 teaspoons of ground cumin
1 tablespoon of low-sodium coconut aminos
1 teaspoon of dried oregano
1 teaspoon of sea salt
1 tablespoon of freshly squeezed lime juice
1/2 cup of sauerkraut
1/4 cup of fresh cilantro, chopped
Instructions:
1.   Press the "Sauté" on your Instant Pot and add the ground beef. Cook until brown.
2.   Season with dried oregano, sea salt, ground cumin, and coconut aminos.
3.   Cover and seal the lid. Press the "Manual" button and cook for 10 minutes at High Pressure.
4.   When the cooking is done, naturally release the pressure and remove the lid. Carefully remove the lid. If there's still any liquid use the "Sauté" function to boil until fully evaporated.
5.   In a large bowl, add the ground beef and the remaining ingredients. Stir until fully combined. Serve and enjoy!
Nutrition information per serving:
- Calories: 333
- Fat: 26g
- Carbohydrates: 10g
- Protein: 21g
- Dietary Fiber: 5g

Meat Recipes

Fit for a King Creamy Ground Beef Sweet Potato Stew

Time: 15 minutes
Servings: 6
Ingredients:

- 2 tablespoons of olive oil
- 2 pounds of grass-fed lean ground beef
- 1 or 2 large sweet potatoes, peeled and cut into 1/2-inch pieces
- 2 cups of homemade low-sodium chicken broth or bone broth
- 3 medium shallots, sliced
- 8-ounces of spinach
- 6 garlic cloves, minced
- 1 tablespoon of dried thyme
- 1 bay leaf
- 1 teaspoon of sea salt
- 1 teaspoon of freshly cracked black pepper

Instructions:

- Press the "Saute" function on your Instant Pot and add the olive oil.
- Once the oil is hot and ready, add the shallots and sauté until lightly golden, stirring occasionally.
- Add the garlic and cook for an additional minute.
- Add the ground beef, dried thyme, salt, and black pepper to your Instant Pot. Cook until brown, stirring occasionally.
- Gently stir in the remaining ingredients except for the spinach.
- Cover and seal the lid on your Instant Pot. Press the "Manual" button and cook for 8 minutes at High Pressure.
- When the cooking is done, manually release the pressure and remove the lid.
- Stir in the spinach and allow to wilt. Adjust the seasoning if necessary.
- Serve and enjoy!

Nutrition information per serving:

- Calories: 402
- Fat: 14.3g
- Carbohydrates: 19g
- Protein: 47.5g
- Dietary Fiber: 2.2g

Rockstar Balsamic Apple Pork Chops

Time: 43 minutes
Servings: 4
Ingredients:
3 pork chops
1/2 medium-sized onions, finely chopped
1 medium-sized apple, peeled, cored, and finely chopped
2 tablespoons of ghee or coconut oil
1 teaspoon of garlic powder
1/2 teaspoon of sea salt
1/2 teaspoon of freshly cracked black pepper
1/3 cup of balsamic vinegar
Instructions:
1.   Press the "Sauté" function on your Instant Pot and add the ghee or coconut oil.
2.   Once hot and ready, add the pork chops and cook for 1 to 2 minutes per side or until brown.
3.   Turn off the "Sauté" function and add the remaining ingredients on top of the pork chops.
4.   Lock the lid and ensure the pressure valve is closed.
5.   Select the "Manual" function and cook for 10 minutes at High Pressure.
6.   When the cooking is done, quick release the pressure and remove the lid.
7.   Remove the pork chops and spread the balsamic/apple mixture over the pork chops.
8.   Serve and enjoy!
Nutrition information per serving:
- Calories: 287
- Fat: 21.4g
- Carbohydrates: 9.2g
- Protein: 13.8g
- Dietary Fiber: 1.6g

To-Die-For Ground Beef Stroganoff

Time: 21 minutes
Servings: 4
Ingredients:
1 pound of grass-fed ground beef
1/2 medium-sized onion, finely chopped
2 garlic cloves, minced
1 cup of cremini mushrooms, sliced
2 tablespoons of coconut flour
1 cup of homemade low-sodium chicken broth
2 teaspoons of low-sodium coconut aminos
1/3 cup of unsweetened coconut cream
1/2 teaspoon of sea salt
1/2 teaspoon of freshly cracked black pepper
Instructions:
1.   Press the "Sauté" function on your Instant Pot and add the olive oil.
2.   Once the oil is hot and ready, add the onions. Sauté until translucent, stirring occasionally.
3.   Add the garlic and sauté for an additional minute.
4.   Add the ground beef and cook until almost brown. Turn off "Sauté" setting.
5.   Add the mushrooms, salt, black pepper, and chicken broth to your Instant Pot.
6.   Lock and seal the lid. Press the "Manual" button and cook for 8 minutes at High Pressure.
7.   When the cooking is done, naturally release the pressure for 5 minutes and then quick release the remaining pressure. Carefully remove the lid.
8.   Gently stir in the coconut cream and adjust the seasoning if necessary.
9.   Serve and enjoy!
Nutrition information per serving:
- Calories: 298
- Fat: 12.7g
- Carbohydrates: 8.6g
- Protein: 36.7g
- Dietary Fiber: 3.9g

Immersive Cranberry Creamy Beef Chili

Time: 25 minutes
Servings: 8
Ingredients:
1 pound of grass-fed lean beef
1 large sweet potato, cut into bite-sized chunks
1 to 2 parsnips, cut into bite-sized chunks
1/4 cup of fresh ginger, peeled and minced
1/4 cup of pure maple syrup
2 cups of leeks, sliced
2 cups of fresh cranberries
5 cups of homemade low-sodium beef broth
1 teaspoon of sea salt
1/2 teaspoon of freshly cracked black pepper
Instructions:
1.   Press the "Sauté" function on your Instant Pot and add the ground beef. Cook until lightly brown, breaking apart as you cook.
2.   Add the remaining ingredients to your Instant Pot and gently stir.
3.   Lock the lid and ensure the valve is closed. Press the "Manual" button and cook for 8 minutes at High Pressure.
4.   When the cooking is done, naturally release the pressure for 5 minutes before quick releasing the remaining pressure. Carefully remove the lid.
5.   Transfer half of the chili to a blender or food processor. Blend until smooth and return to your Instant Pot.
6.   Give a good stir and adjust the seasoning if necessary.
7.   Serve and enjoy!
Nutrition information per serving:
- Calories: 207
- Fat: 3.9g
- Carbohydrates: 23.1g
- Protein: 3.8g
- Dietary Fiber: 18.5g.

Dreamy Beef Goulash

Time: 30 minutes
Servings: 4
Ingredients:
2 pounds of beef roast or stew meat, cut into 1-inch pieces
1 cup of white button mushrooms, quartered
2 medium-sized carrots, cut into 1-inch pieces
4 tablespoons of olive oil
1 medium-sized onions, peeled and chopped
4 garlic cloves, minced
1 teaspoon of turmeric
1 cup of homemade low-sodium bone broth
1 tablespoon of coconut flour
2 tablespoons of fresh parsley, finely chopped
1 teaspoon of sea salt
1 teaspoon of freshly cracked black pepper
Instructions:
1.   Press the "Sauté" function on your Instant Pot and add the olive oil.
2.   Once the oil is hot and ready, add the ground beef and cook until brown.
3.   Add the onions and garlic to your Instant Pot and cook for an additional minute.
4.   Add the mushrooms, carrots, turmeric, salt, black pepper, and bone broth to your Instant Pot.
5.   Close and seal the lid on your Instant Pot. Press the "Manual" button and cook for 20 minutes at High Pressure.
6.   When the cooking is done, naturally release the pressure for 10 minutes before manually releasing the rest of the pressure. Carefully remove the lid.
7.   Press the "Sauté" function on your Instant Pot and sprinkle the coconut flour and fresh parsley over. Cook until the liquid thickens and adjusts the seasoning if necessary.
8.   Serve and enjoy!
Nutrition information per serving:
- Calories: 449
- Fat: 14.2g
- Carbohydrates: 6.3g
- Protein: 69.9g
- Dietary Fiber: 1.5g

Yearlong Turkey Chili

Time: 25 minutes
Servings: 6
Ingredients:
1 pound of lean ground turkey
1 medium-sized onion, finely chopped
1 cup of organic pureed pumpkin
1 cup of zucchini, finely chopped
1 tablespoon of freshly squeezed lemon juice
1/2 cup of fresh green onions, finely chopped
1 cup of carrots, finely chopped
1/2 cup of celery, finely chopped
2 cups of homemade low-sodium chicken broth or vegetable broth
2 tablespoons of olive oil
1 teaspoon of sea salt
1 teaspoon of garlic powder
1 teaspoon of ground cumin
1/2 teaspoon of turmeric
1/2 teaspoon of dried oregano
1 teaspoon of freshly cracked black pepper
Instructions:
1.   In a small bowl, add the sea salt, ground cumin, turmeric, dried oregano, garlic powder and freshly cracked black pepper. Mix well.
2.   Press the "Sauté" function on your Instant Pot and add the ground turkey. Cook until lightly browned, breaking apart as you cook.
3.   Add the vegetables and cook for 4 to 6 minutes.
4.   Add the remaining ingredients including the organic pureed pumpkin.
5.   Cover and seal the lid. Press the "Manual" button and cook for 5 minutes at High Pressure.
6.   When the cooking is done, naturally release the pressure for 10 minutes before quick releasing the remaining pressure. Carefully remove the lid.
7.   Serve and enjoy!
Nutrition information per serving:
- Calories: 221
- Fat: 13.2g
- Carbohydrates: 7.7g
- Protein: 2.4g
- Dietary Fiber: 21.8g

Forever Bacon Maple Balsamic Pulled Pork

Time: 1 hour and 30 minutes
Servings: 8

Ingredients:

4 pounds of pork shoulder roast, trimmed and cut into 3 large separate pieces
1/2 medium-sized onion, sliced
6 medium-sized bacon slices
1/4 cup of balsamic vinegar
2 teaspoons of fish sauce
2 teaspoons of sea salt
1 teaspoon of garlic powder
2 tablespoons of pure maple syrup
1 teaspoon of organic ground cinnamon powder
1 cup of homemade low-sodium bone broth

Instructions:

1. In a bowl, add the sea salt, ground cinnamon powder, and garlic powder. Mix well.
2. Rub the spice mixture over the pork pieces and place to the bottom of your Instant Pot.
3. Lay the bacon slices on top along with the onions.
4. Pour the balsamic vinegar, bone broth, and fish sauce over the pork.
5. Close and seal the lid. Press the "Manual" button and cook for 1 hour and 40 minutes.
6. When the cooking is done, naturally release the pressure and remove the lid.
7. Transfer the roast, onion, and bacon to a cutting board and shred using two forks.
8. In a medium bowl, add ½ cup of cooking liquid from inside your Instant Pot and 2 tablespoons of pure maple syrup. Mix well.
9. Combine the mixture with the pulled pork.
10. Serve and enjoy!

Nutrition information per serving:

- Calories: 431
- Fat: 13.9g
- Carbohydrates: 7.5g
- Protein: 64.7g
- Dietary Fiber: 0.2g

Crazy Loaded Sweet Potatoes with Pulled Pork

Time: 1 hour
Servings: 4
Ingredients:
1-1/2 pounds of pork roast
2 tablespoons of coconut oil
1 small onion, finely chopped
1 small apple, cored, peeled, and finely chopped
1 cup of kale, roughly chopped
2 tablespoons of apple cider vinegar
4 medium-sized bacon slices, cooked and chopped
2 teaspoons of fresh ginger, minced
2 garlic cloves, minced
1 cup of water
1 teaspoon of turmeric
1/2 teaspoon of organic ground cinnamon
1/2 teaspoon of sea salt
1/4 cup of fresh cilantro, finely chopped
Instructions:
1.   Press the "Sauté" function on your Instant Pot and add the coconut oil.
2.   Once the oil is hot, add the pork and cook for 5 minutes.
3.   Lock the lid and ensure the valve is closed. Press the "Manual" button and cook for 50 minutes at High Pressure.
4.   Meanwhile, you can prepare you can cook your bacon until brown and crispy. Set aside.
5.   When the cooking is done, allow for a 5-minute natural release method before manually releasing the rest of the pressure.
6.   In a bowl, add the finely chopped onion, finely chopped apple, water, apple cider vinegar, minced ginger, minced garlic, turmeric, cinnamon, and sea salt. Mix well.
7.   Pour the spice mixture over the pork roast.
8.   Transfer the pork to a cutting board and shred using two forks. Stir in the fresh cilantro.
9.   To prepare the stuffed sweet potatoes, cut each potato half lengthwise and scoop out inner portions.
10.   Divide the pork combination among the 4 sweet potatoes and top with kale and bacon.
11.   Place the sweet potatoes on top of the baking dish and bake for 20 minutes at 350 degrees Fahrenheit.
12.   Serve and enjoy!
Nutrition information per serving:
*   Calories: 463
*   Fat: 20.9g
*   Carbohydrates: 12.1g
*   Protein: 52.1g
*   Dietary Fiber: 2.1g

Agreeable Roasted Lemon Beef

Time: 20 minutes

Servings: 4

Ingredients:

2 pounds of grass-fed ground beef

2 tablespoons of ghee or coconut oil

1 medium-sized onion, finely chopped

4 garlic cloves, minced

1 medium-sized lemon, juice

2 teaspoons of sea salt

1 teaspoon of freshly cracked black pepper

Instructions:

1.   Press the "Sauté" function on your Instant Pot and add the ghee.
2.   Once hot, add the onions and cook until translucent, stirring occasionally.
3.   Add the garlic and cook for an additional minute.
4.   Add the ground beef and cook until mostly brown, stirring occasionally.
5.   Add the lemon juice, sea salt, and freshly cracked black pepper.
6.   Lock the lid and ensure the valve is closed. Press the "Manual" button and cook for 8 minutes at High Pressure.
7.   When the cooking is done, naturally release the pressure for 5 minutes and then quick release the remaining pressure. Carefully remove the lid.
8.   Serve and enjoy!

Nutrition information per serving:

- Calories: 502
- Fat: 21g
- Carbohydrates: 5.5g
- Protein: 69.5g
- Dietary Fiber: 1.2g

Poultry Recipes

Spectacular Chicken Liver with Onions

Time: 20 minutes
Servings: 4
Ingredients:
1 bag of chicken livers
1 large onion, finely chopped
1 tablespoon of coconut oil
3 garlic cloves, minced
1 to 2 cups of homemade low-sodium chicken broth
2 tablespoons of coconut flour
1 tablespoon of fresh parsley, finely chopped
1 tablespoon of fresh rosemary, chopped
1 teaspoon of sea salt
1 teaspoon of freshly cracked black pepper
Instructions:
1.	Press the "Sauté" function on your Instant Pot and add the coconut oil.
2.	Once the oil is hot, add the chicken livers, onion, and garlic. Sauté for about 3 to 4 minutes or until softened, stirring occasionally
3.	Add the chicken broth to your Instant Pot.
4.	Close and seal the lid. Press the "Manual" button and cook for 10 minutes at High Pressure.
5.	When the cooking is done, naturally release the pressure for 5 minutes before quick releasing the rest of the pressure.
6.	Press the "Sauté" function on your Instant Pot and sprinkle with coconut flour. Allow the liquid to thicken.
7.	Season with sea salt and freshly cracked black pepper. Garnish with fresh parsley and fresh rosemary.
8.	Serve and enjoy!
Nutrition information per serving:
- Calories: 264
- Fat: 11.6g
- Carbohydrates: 9.5g
- Protein: 29.3g
- Dietary Fiber: 3.8g

Amazingly Tasty Turmeric Chicken

Time: 20 minutes
Servings: 6
Ingredients:
2 pounds of boneless skinless chicken thighs or chicken breasts
2 cups of fresh celery, finely chopped
2 cups of fresh carrots, finely chopped
1 cup of yellow onions, finely chopped
3 tablespoons of coconut oil or olive oil
2 teaspoons of sea salt
1 teaspoon of freshly cracked black pepper
1 teaspoon of turmeric
4 cups of homemade low-sodium chicken broth or chicken stock
Instructions:
1.   Press the "Sauté" function on your Instant Pot and add the coconut oil.
2.   Once the oil is hot and ready, add the onions and cook for 3 to 5 minutes or until softened.
3.   Add the celery and carrots to your Instant Pot and season with salt, turmeric, and black pepper.
4.   Place the chicken on top of the vegetables and pour in the chicken stock.
5.   Lock the lid and ensure the valve is closed. Press the "Manual" button and cook for 15 minutes at High Pressure.
6.   When your Instant Pot timer beeps, manually release the pressure and remove the lid.
7.   Transfer the chicken to a cutting board and shred using two forks. Return to your Instant Pot and give a good stir. Adjust the seasoning if necessary.
8.   Serve and enjoy!
Nutrition information per serving:
- Calories: 341
- Fat: 12.6g
- Carbohydrates: 7g
- Protein: 47.8g
- Dietary Fiber: 1.9g

Defining 40-Garlic Clove Chicken

Time: 30 minutes
Servings: 6

6 bone-in, skin-on chicken thighs or chicken breasts
2 tablespoons of coconut oil
1 teaspoon of sea salt
1 teaspoon of freshly cracked black pepper
1 cup of garlic cloves, peeled
1/4 cup of dry white wine
1/4 cup of homemade low-sodium chicken broth
2 fresh sprigs of thyme
Instructions:
1.   Season the chicken with sea salt and black pepper.
2.   Press the "Sauté" function on your Instant Pot and add the coconut oil.
3.   Once the oil is hot, working in batches, add the chicken and cook for 2 to 3 minutes per side or until brown. Remove and set aside.
4.   Add the garlic and fresh sprigs of thyme to your Instant Pot. Give a good stir and cook for 1 minute.
5.   Turn off the "Sauté" setting and add in the dry white wine and chicken broth.
6.   Return the chicken breasts or thighs to your Instant Pot.
7.   Lock the lid and ensure the valve is closed. Press the "Manual" button and cook for 15 minutes at High Pressure.
8.   When the cooking is done, naturally release the pressure for 5 minutes before quick releasing the resto f the pressure. Carefully remove the lid.
9.   Serve and enjoy!
Nutrition information per serving:
- Calories: 326
- Fat: 15.4g
- Carbohydrates: 0.3g
- Protein: 42.5g
- Dietary Fiber: 0g

Desirable Filipino-Inspired Adobo Chicken

Time: 25 minutes
Servings: 6
Ingredients:
6 bone-in, skin on chicken legs
1 garlic head, peeled and smashed
1 medium-sized onions, sliced
4 bay leaves
1/2 cup of homemade low-sodium chicken broth or chicken stock
2/3 cup of low-sodium coconut aminos
2/3 cup of apple cider vinegar
1 teaspoon of fish sauce
1 teaspoon of sea salt
2 teaspoons of freshly cracked black pepper
Instructions:
1.	In a bowl, add the coconut aminos, apple cider vinegar, chicken broth, fish sauce, sea salt, and black pepper. Mix well.
2.	Add the chicken legs, smashed garlic cloves, 4 bay leaves, and onions to your Instant Pot.
3.	Pour the liquid mixture over.
4.	Lock the lid and ensure the valve is closed. Press the "Manual" button and cook for 18 minutes at High Pressure.
5.	When the cooking is done, quick release the pressure and remove the lid.
6.	Remove the chicken legs and sliced onions from your Instant Pot.
7.	Discard the 4 bay leaves.
8.	Press the "Sauté" function on your Instant Pot and cook until the liquid thickens, stirring occasionally.
9.	Ladle the sauce over the chicken legs.
10.	Serve and enjoy!
Nutrition information per serving:
- Calories: 308
- Fat: 10.9g
- Carbohydrates: 5.6g
- Protein: 42.7g
- Dietary Fiber: 0.6g

Lovely Pumpkin Enchilada Chicken

Time: 36 minutes
Servings: 4
Ingredients:
2 pounds of boneless, skinless chicken breasts
2 tablespoons of olive oil
1 medium-sized sweet onions, finely chopped
2 garlic cloves, minced
2 cups of organic pureed pumpkin
1 cup of Nomato sauce or any other AIP alternative tomato sauces
1/2 teaspoon of ground cumin
1 teaspoon of sea salt
Instructions:
1.   Season the chicken breasts with sea salt.
2.   Press the "Sauté" function on your Instant Pot and add the olive oil.
3.   Once the oil is hot, add the chicken breasts and cook for 4 minutes on both sides or until brown. Remove and set aside.
4.   Add the onions and garlic to your Instant Pot and sauté until translucent, stirring occasionally.
5.   Add the pureed pumpkin, nomato sauce, ground cumin to your Instant Pot. Give a good stir.
6.   Return the chicken to your Instant Pot.
7.   Lock the lid and ensure the valve is closed. Press the "Manual" button and cook for 12 minutes at High Pressure.
8.   When the cooking is done, allow for a 10 minute naturally release before quick releasing the rest of the pressure. Carefully remove the lid.
9.   Transfer the chicken to a cutting board and shred using two forks. Return the chicken to your Instant Pot and stir until well coated with the sauce.
10.   Press the "Sauté" function on your Instant Pot and cook until some of the liquid has reduced.
11.   Serve and enjoy!
Nutrition information per serving:
- Calories: 479
- Fat: 14.4g
- Carbohydrates: 18.2g
- Protein: 68.2g
- Dietary Fiber: 6g

Luxurious White Chicken Chili

Time: 25 minutes
Servings: 8
Ingredients:
4 boneless skinless chicken breasts or chicken thighs
1 to 2 large white yams, cut into 1/2-inch pieces
4 medium-sized celery stalks, chopped
4 medium-sized carrots, chopped
1 medium yellow onion, finely chopped
3 garlic cloves, minced
1 teaspoon of ground cumin
1/4 teaspoon of dried oregano
1/2 teaspoon of garlic powder
1/2 teaspoon of onion powder
2 teaspoons of sea salt
1 cup of unsweetened coconut milk
2 cups of homemade low-sodium chicken broth
2 medium-sized avocados, ripe, peeled and chopped (topping)
4 green onions, sliced (topping)
Instructions:
1.   Add all the ingredients except for the avocados and the green onions to your Instant Pot.
2.   Close and seal the lid. Press the "Manual" button and cook for 20 minutes at High Pressure.
3.   When the cooking is done, quick release the pressure and carefully remove the lid.
4.   Transfer the chicken breasts or chicken thighs to a cutting board. Shred using two forks.
5.   Return the shredded chicken to your Instant Pot.
Ladle the chili into serving bowls and top with desired toppings.
6.   Serve and enjoy!
Nutrition information per serving:
- Calories: 407
- Fat: 22.8g
- Carbohydrates: 26.8g
- Protein: 25.4g
- Dietary Fiber: 7.5g

Soulfully Apple Shredded Chicken

Time: 25 minutes
Servings: 4
Ingredients:
4 boneless, skinless chicken breasts or chicken thighs
4 medium-sized bacon slices, finely chopped
1 cup of apples, finely chopped
1/2 cup of unsweetened coconut milk
1/2 cup of homemade low-sodium chicken broth
1/2 teaspoon of sea salt
Instructions:
1.   Press the "Sauté" function on your Instant Pot and add the bacon. Cook until brown and crispy, stirring occasionally.
2.   Turn off the "Sauté" setting and remove the bacon. Transfer to a plate lined with paper towels.
3.   In a blender, add the chicken broth, unsweetened coconut milk, salt, and ½ cup of chopped apples. Blend until smooth.
4.   Return the bacon, chicken breast, and remaining chopped apple to your Instant Pot.
5.   Pour the apple mixture over the chicken.
6.   Cover and seal the lid. Press the "Manual" button and cook for 20 minutes at High Pressure.
7.   When the cooking is done, quick release the pressure and remove the lid.
8.   Transfer the chicken breast to a cutting board and shred using two forks.
9.   Return the shredded chicken to your Instant Pot and combine with the mixture.
10.   Serve and enjoy!
Nutrition information per serving:
- Calories: 483
- Fat: 26.3g
- Carbohydrates: 9.7g
- Protein: 50.7g
- Dietary Fiber:2g

Family Favorite Chicken and Mushrooms

Time: 30 minutes
Servings: 4
Ingredients:
2 pounds of boneless, skinless chicken breasts or chicken thighs
2 tablespoons of olive oil or coconut oil
1 large onion, finely chopped
2 garlic cloves, minced
2 cups of cremini mushrooms, sliced
1 bay leaf
2 fresh sprigs of rosemary
2 tablespoons of red wine vinegar
1 to 2 tablespoons of coconut flour
1/2 cup of unsweetened coconut cream
2 teaspoons of sea salt
1/2 teaspoon of ground nutmeg
1 teaspoon of garlic powder
Instructions:
1.   Press the "Sauté" function on your Instant Pot and add the olive oil or coconut oil.
2.   Once the oil is hot, add the chopped onion, minced garlic, and bay leaf to your Instant Pot. Sauté for 8 to 10 minutes or until softened, stirring occasionally.
3.   Add the sliced mushrooms and fresh sprigs of rosemary to your Instant Pot. Cook for another 5 minutes or until tender, stirring occasionally.
4.   Season the chicken thighs with sea salt and add to your Instant Pot. Cook until mostly brown on both sides.
5.   Add the red wine vinegar and give a good stir.
6.   Add in ¼ cup of unsweetened coconut cream and turn off the "Sauté" setting.
7.   Lock the lid and ensure the valve is sealed. Press the "Manual" button and cook for 10 minutes at High Pressure.
8.   When the cooking is done, quick release the pressure and carefully remove the lid.
9.   Transfer the chicken to a cutting board and shred using two forks. Return to your Instant Pot.
10.   Press the "Sauté" function on your Instant Pot. Stir in the remaining ¼ cup of unsweetened coconut cream along with the coconut flour. Allow simmering until smooth.
11.   Serve and enjoy!
Nutrition information per serving:
- Calories: 616
- Fat: 31.9g
- Carbohydrates: 11.9g
- Protein: 4.8g
- Dietary Fiber: 68.9g

Important Mango Chicken

Time: 33 minutes
Servings: 4
Ingredients:
4 boneless, skinless chicken breasts or chicken thighs, cut into bite-sized pieces
3 cups of fresh mango cubes
4 garlic cloves, minced
1 tablespoon of fresh ginger, peeled and finely minced
1/2 cup of unsweetened coconut milk
2 tablespoons of low-sodium coconut aminos
1 tablespoon of apple cider vinegar
1 teaspoon of turmeric
1 teaspoon of sea salt
Instructions:
1.   In a blender, add the mango cubes, minced garlic, minced ginger, coconut milk, coconut aminos, apple cider vinegar, turmeric, and sea salt. Blend until smooth.
2.   Add the chicken pieces to your Instant Pot and pour in the mango sauce.
3.   Lock the lid and ensure the valve is closed. Press the "Manual" button and cook for 15 minutes at High Pressure.
4.   When the cooking is done, allow for a full natural release and carefully remove the lid.
5.   Serve and enjoy!
Nutrition information per serving:
- Calories: 430
- Fat: 18.5g
- Carbohydrates: 22.2g
- Protein: 44.2g
- Dietary Fiber: 2.7g

Occasional Shredded Chicken with Kale and Tarragon

Time: 23 minutes
Servings: 6
Ingredients:
6 boneless, skinless chicken thighs or chicken breasts
2 tablespoons of coconut oil
1 large leek, thinly sliced
4 garlic cloves, minced
2 to 4 teaspoons of dried tarragon
1 cup of homemade low-sodium chicken broth
1 large bunch of kale, roughly chopped
3/4 cup of organic pureed pumpkin
2 teaspoons of sea salt
Instructions:
1. Add the chicken thighs and ½ cup of homemade low-sodium chicken broth to your Instant Pot.
2. Lock the lid and ensure the valve is sealed. Press the "Manual" button and cook for 15 minutes at High Pressure.
3. When the cooking is done, manually release the pressure and remove the lid.
4. Transfer the chicken to a cutting board and shred using two forks. Discard the liquid from your Instant Pot.
5. Press the "Sauté" function on your Instant Pot and add the coconut oil.
6. Once the oil is hot, add the sliced leeks. Sauté for 4 minutes or until slightly softened, stirring occasionally.
7. Add the minced garlic, dried tarragon, pureed pumpkin, and remaining ½ cup of homemade low-sodium chicken broth to your Instant Pot. Allow simmering until thickened.
8. Return the shredded chicken with the roughly chopped kale to your Instant Pot. Cook until the kale wilts down.
9. Season with salt.
10. Serve and enjoy!
Nutrition information per serving:
- Calories: 361
- Fat: 15.5g
- Carbohydrates: 9.9g
- Protein: 44.3g
- Dietary Fiber: 1.9g

Very Creamy Chicken Chowder with Bacon

Time: 30 minutes
Servings: 6
Ingredients:
6 boneless, skinless chicken breasts or chicken thighs, cut into bite-sized pieces
1 pound of bacon, finely chopped
2 cups of unsweetened coconut cream
1 large yellow onion, finely chopped
4 garlic cloves, minced
2 celery ribs, finely chopped
1 cup of cremini mushrooms, thinly sliced
2 tablespoons of coconut butter or coconut oil
1 fresh sprig of thyme
1 teaspoon of sea salt
2 cups of fresh spinach or kale
3 cups of homemade low-sodium chicken broth
Instructions:
1.	Press the "Sauté" function on your Instant Pot and add the coconut oil.
2.	When the oil is hot, add the chicken and cook until brown on both sides. Turn off the "Sauté" setting.
3.	Add all the ingredients except for the coconut cream, bacon, and spinach to your Instant Pot and give a good stir.
4.	Lock the lid and ensure the valve is closed. Press the "Manual" button and cook for 30 minutes at High Pressure.
5.	Meanwhile, you can cook your bacon and set aside.
6.	When the cooking is done, naturally release the pressure for 10 minutes before quick releasing the rest of the pressure. Carefully remove the lid.
7.	Stir in the unsweetened coconut cream and spinach. Press the "Sauté" function on your Instant Pot and allow to cook until the spinach has wilted.
8.	Top with the chopped cooked bacon.
9.	Serve and enjoy!
Nutrition information per serving:
•	Calories: 739
•	Fat: 53.5g
•	Carbohydrates: 7.1g
•	Protein: 57.1g
•	Dietary Fiber: 2.1g

Glamourous Curried Coconut and Lemon Chicken

Time: 40 minutes
Servings: 6
Ingredients:
4 pounds of boneless, skinless chicken breasts or chicken thighs
2 cups of broccoli florets
1-1/2 cup of unsweetened coconut milk
1/2 cup of homemade low-sodium chicken broth
1/4 cup of freshly squeezed lemon juice
1 teaspoons of turmeric
1 teaspoon of fresh lemon zest
1/2 teaspoon of sea salt
Instructions:
1.	In a bowl, add the coconut milk, chicken broth, lemon juice, turmeric, lemon zest, and sea salt. Mix well.
2.	Add the chicken and broccoli to your Instant Pot and pour in the coconut mixture.
3.	Lock the lid and ensure the valve is sealed. Press the "Manual" button and cook for 15 minutes at High Pressure.
4.	When the cooking is done, quick release the pressure and carefully remove the lid.
5.	Transfer the chicken to a cutting board and shred using two forks.
6.	Return the shredded chicken to your Instant Pot. Adjust the seasoning if necessary.
7.	Serve and enjoy!
Nutrition information per serving:
- Calories: 725
- Fat: 36.9g
- Carbohydrates: 5.5g
- Protein: 89.8g
- Dietary Fiber: 2.2g

Confident Chicken with Apples, Carrots, and Plums

Time: 25 minutes
Servings: 6
Ingredients:
2 pounds of boneless skinless chicken breasts or chicken thighs
1 pound of carrots, finely chopped
1 large red onion, roughly chopped
2-1/2 apples, peeled, cored, and finely chopped
10 plums, pitted
1-1/2 cup of unsweetened coconut milk
2 teaspoons of sea salt
Instructions:
1.	Add all the ingredients to your Instant Pot and stir until completely combined.
2.	Lock the lid and ensure the valve is closed. Press the "Manual" button and cook for 15 minutes at High Pressure.
3.	When the cooking is done, naturally release the pressure and carefully remove the lid.
4.	Adjust the seasoning if necessary.
5.	Serve and enjoy!
Nutrition information per serving:
- Calories: 506
- Fat: 19.4g
- Carbohydrates: 39.3g
- Protein: 47.2g
- Dietary Fiber: 7.5g

Only the Greatest Ginger-Balsamic Chicken

Time: 30 minutes
Servings: 8
Ingredients:
8 boneless, skinless chicken thighs or chicken breasts
2 to 4 tablespoons of coconut oil
1/3 cup of balsamic vinegar
4 garlic cloves, minced
2 tablespoons of fresh ginger, peeled and minced
4 tablespoons of pure honey
2 teaspoons of sea salt
Instructions:
1.   Press the "Sauté" function on your Instant Pot and add the coconut oil.
2.   Once the oil is hot, working in batches if necessary, add the chicken thighs and cook until brown on both sides.
3.   In a bowl, add the balsamic vinegar, minced garlic, minced ginger, honey, and sea salt. Mix well.
4.   Add the chicken to your Instant Pot and pour the ginger mixture over.
5.   Lock the lid and ensure the valve is closed. Press the "Manual" button and cook for 10 minutes at High Pressure.
6.   When the cooking is done, naturally release the pressure for 10 minutes before quick releasing the rest of the pressure. Carefully remove the lid.
7.   Serve and enjoy!
Nutrition information per serving:
- Calories: 377
- Fat: 17.7g
- Carbohydrates: 10.2g
- Protein: 0.2g
- Dietary Fiber: 42.5g

Considerate Honey Garlic Chicken

Time: 30 minutes
Servings: 4
Ingredients:
6 skin-on, bone-in chicken breasts or chicken thighs
1/2 cup of low-sodium coconut aminos
4 garlic cloves, minced
1 tablespoon of fresh ginger, minced
1/3 cup of raw honey
2 tablespoons of fresh parsley, finely chopped
1 teaspoon of dried oregano
1/4 cup of homemade low-sodium chicken broth
1/2 cup of organic pureed pumpkin
2 tablespoons of coconut flour
2 tablespoons of coconut oil or olive oil
2 teaspoons of sea salt
Instructions:
1.   In a bowl, add the coconut aminos, minced garlic, minced ginger, raw honey, fresh parsley, dried oregano, and pureed pumpkin. Mix until fully combined.
2.   Season the chicken breasts with sea salt.
3.   Press the "Sauté" function on your Instant Pot and add the coconut oil.
4.   Once the oil is hot, working in batches if necessary, add the chicken breasts and cook until brown on both sides.
5.   Add the honey mixture over the chicken.
6.   Lock the lid and ensure the valve is closed. Press the "Manual" button and cook for 20 minutes at High Pressure.
7.   When the cooking is done, naturally release the pressure for 5 minutes before quick releasing the remaining pressure. Carefully remove the lid.
8.   Transfer the chicken to a plate and ladle the honey sauce over.
9.   Serve and enjoy!
Nutrition information per serving:
- Calories: 363
- Fat: 12.2g
- Carbohydrates: 29g
- Protein: 34.3g
- Dietary Fiber: 5g

Fish and Seafood Recipes

Notable Greek Grilled Octopus

Time: 22 minutes
Servings: 6
Ingredients:
2 pounds of octopus, cleaned
1/2 medium-sized lemon
3 tablespoons of coconut oil or olive oil
1/2 red onion, thinly sliced
2 fresh sprigs of rosemary
4 fresh sprigs of thyme
2 teaspoons of dried oregano
1 teaspoon of sea salt
Marinade Ingredients:
1.   1/4 cup of olive oil
2.   2 tablespoons of freshly squeezed lemon juice
3.   4 garlic cloves, minced
4.   1 fresh sprig of rosemary
5.   2 fresh sprigs of thyme
6.   1 teaspoon of sea salt
7.   Instructions:
8.   Add the cleaned octopus, lemon, coconut oil, red onion, rosemary, thyme, dried oregano, and sea salt to your Instant Pot.
9.   Lock the lid and ensure the valve is closed. Press the "Manual" button and cook at Low for 10 minutes.
10.   When the cooking is done, naturally release the pressure and carefully remove the lid.
11.   Transfer the octopus to a cutting board and cut into bite-sized pieces
12.   In a large bowl, add all the marinade ingredients and mix well.
13.   Brush the marinade over the octopus.
14.   Preheat your grill on High and add the octopus. Grill until lightly charred or reached your desired texture.
15.   Serve and enjoy!
Nutrition information per serving:
- Calories: 213
- Fat: 10.2g
- Carbohydrates: 4.2g
- Protein: 25.4g
- Dietary Fiber: 0.1g

Marathon Chinese-Inspired Ginger Fish

Time: 25 minutes
Servings: 4
Ingredients:
1 pound of tilapia fish
1 tablespoon of coconut oil.
2 garlic cloves, minced
1 teaspoon of fresh ginger, minced
2 tablespoons of low-sodium coconut aminos
2 tablespoons of dry white wine
1/4 cup of green onions, julienned
1/4 cup of fresh cilantro, chopped
Instructions:
1.   In a bowl, add the minced garlic, minced ginger, coconut aminos, and dry white wine. Mix well.
2.   Add the tilapia fish to the marinade. Allow marinating for 30 minutes to 1 hour.
3.   Add 2 cups of water and a steamer rack to your Instant Pot.
4.   Place the tilapia fish on the steamer rack. Reserve the marinade for later use.
5.   Lock the lid and ensure the valve is closed. Press the "Manual" button and cook at Low for 2 minutes.
6.   When the cooking is done, quick release the pressure and carefully remove the lid.
7.   In a saucepan over medium-high heat, add the coconut oil. Add the reserved marinade and allow to simmer until heated through.
8.   Pour the marinade over the tilapia fish.
9.   Serve and enjoy!
Nutrition information per serving:
- Calories: 173
- Fat: 6g
- Carbohydrates: 5g
- Protein: 26g
- Dietary Fiber: 2.32g

Excitable Honey Garlicky Shrimp

Time: 20 minutes
Servings: 4
Ingredients:
1 pound of shrimp, peeled and deveined
1 tablespoon of coconut oil
8 garlic cloves, minced
1 tablespoon of fresh ginger, peeled and minced
1/4 cup of low-sodium coconut aminos
1/4 cup of raw honey
Instructions:
1.   In a bowl, add the coconut aminos, honey, ginger, and garlic. Mix well.
2.   Add shrimp to your Instant Pot along with the marinade and coconut oil.
3.   Lock the lid and ensure the valve is closed. Press the "Manual" button and cook at High Pressure for 5 minutes.
4.   When the cooking is done, quick release the pressure and carefully remove the lid.
5.   Allow the sauce to thicken and gently stir until fully coated.
6.   Serve and enjoy!
Nutrition information per serving:
- Calories: 210
- Fat: 5g
- Carbohydrates: 21.32g
- Protein: 26.3g
- Dietary Fiber: 2g

Glorious Lemon Salmon

Time: 20 minutes
Servings: 4
Ingredients:
1 pound of skin-on salmon fillets
1 cup of water
1 tablespoon of fresh parsley, finely chopped
2 tablespoons of coconut oil
1 medium-sized zucchini, julienned
1 large carrot, julienned
1 medium-sized lemon, thinly sliced
1 teaspoon of sea salt
Instructions:
1.   Add 1 cup of water and a steamer rack to your Instant Pot.
2.   Place the salmon fillets on the steamer rack.
3.   Drizzle with 1 tablespoon of coconut oil.
4.   Season with sea salt and top with lemon slices.
5.   Lock the lid and ensure the valve is sealed. Press the "Steam" setting and set the time to 3 minutes. Press start.
6.   When your Instant Pot beeps, quick release the pressure and carefully remove the lid.
7.   Transfer the salmon to a plate.
8.   Discard the liquid from your Instant Pot along with the steamer rack.
9.   Press the "Sauté" function on your Instant Pot and add the coconut oil.
10.   Once hot, add the julienned zucchini and julienned carrots. Sauté for 2 minutes and turn off the "Sauté" function on your Instant Pot.
11.   Add the vegetables to a plate with salmon and garnish with fresh parsley.
12.   Serve and enjoy!
Nutrition information per serving:
- Calories: 224
- Fat: 13.9g
- Carbohydrates: 3.4g
- Protein: 22.8g
- Dietary Fiber: 1g

Kind Tilapia Fish Packets

Time: 15 minutes
Servings: 4
Ingredients:
1 pound of tilapia fish fillets
1 cup of medium zucchini, finely chopped
1 tablespoon of capers, drained
3 garlic cloves, minced
4 tablespoons of freshly squeezed lemon juice
1 cup of water
1 teaspoon of sea salt
Instructions:
1.   Add 1 cup of water and a trivet to your Instant Pot.
2.   Season tilapia fish fillets with sea salt and place on tin foil.
3.   Squeeze the lemon juice and add the zucchini, capers, and garlic cloves.
4.   Fold the tin foil packets together to create a packet.
5.   Place the packet on top of the trivet.
6.   Lock the lid and ensure the valve is sealed. Press the "Manual" button and cook at High Pressure for 5 minutes.
7.   When the cooking is done, quick release the pressure and carefully remove the lid.
8.   Remove the fish packets from your Instant Pot and unfold the packet.
9.   Serve and enjoy!
Nutrition information per serving:
- Calories: 102
- Fat: 1.2g
- Carbohydrates: 1.4g
- Protein: 21.6g
- Dietary Fiber: 0.4g

Restful Herbed Salmon Fillets with Mushrooms and Spinach

Time: 10 minutes

Servings: 4

Ingredients:

1 pound of salmon

2 cups of mushrooms, finely chopped

2 cups of zucchini, finely chopped

2 cups of spinach, roughly chopped

3/4 cups of fresh basil, finely chopped

3/4 cups of fresh parsley, finely chopped

3 garlic cloves, minced

3 tablespoons of coconut oil

1/2 teaspoon of fresh zest

1/4 cup of freshly squeezed lime juice

1 teaspoon of sea salt

1 cup of water

Instructions:

1.   In a bowl, add the zucchini, mushrooms, and spinach. Stir until combined.

2.   In a food processor, add the fresh basil, fresh parsley, minced garlic, coconut oil, fresh lime zest, and sea salt. Pulse until smooth.

3.   Divide the salmon between aluminum foil pieces and pour the herb mixture over until fully coated.

4.   Top each salmon with the vegetable combination.

5.   Tightly fold the aluminum foil to create a packet.

6.   Add 1 cup of water and a trivet to your Instant Pot.

7.   Place the foil on top of the trivet. Lock the lid and ensure the valve is closed. Press the "Manual" button and cook for 5 minutes at High Pressure.

8.   When the cooking is done, quick release the pressure and carefully remove the lid.

9.   Carefully take out the fish packets from your Instant Pot and unfold.

10.   Serve and enjoy!

Nutrition information per serving:

- Calories: 256
- Fat: 15g
- Carbohydrates: 9g
- Protein: 27g
- Dietary Fiber: 3.2g

Talented Garlic "Butter" Salmon

Time: 10 minutes
Servings: 4
Ingredients:
1 pound of salmon fillets, cut into 3 equal-sized pieces
1 pound of asparagus, trimmed
1/4 cup of freshly squeezed lemon juice
4 tablespoons of coconut butter or ghee
4 garlic cloves, finely minced
1 teaspoon of sea salt
1 cup of water
Instructions:
1.	Prepare 3 large pieces of aluminum foil and place on a flat surface.
2.	Divide the asparagus among the foil.
3.	Season the salmon fillets with sea salt and place above the asparagus.
4.	Top with minced garlic and coconut butter.
5.	Tightly wrap the foil to create a packet.
6.	Add 1 cup of water and a steamer rack to your Instant Pot.
7.	Place the salmon packet on top of the steamer rack.
8.	Lock the lid and ensure the valve is sealed. Press the "Steam" setting and adjust the time to 4 minutes. Press "Start".
9.	When your Instant Pot beeps, quick release the pressure and carefully remove the lid.
10.	Carefully remove the salmon packets and unfold.
11.	Serve and enjoy!
Nutrition information per serving:
- Calories: 367
- Fat: 25.3g
- Carbohydrates: 12.7g
- Protein: 26.8g
- Dietary Fiber: 7.5g

Gourmet Honey Balsamic Salmon

Time: 5 minutes
Servings: 4
Ingredients:
4 (5-ounce) pieces of boneless salmon fillets
4 tablespoons of balsamic vinegar
4 tablespoons of raw honey
1 teaspoon of sea salt
1 cup of water
Instructions:
1.	Season each salmon fillet with sea salt.
2.	In a bowl, add the balsamic vinegar and honey. Mix well.
3.	Generously brush the balsamic vinegar/honey mixture over each salmon fillet.
4.	Add 1 cup of water and a trivet to your Instant Pot.
5.	Lock the lid and ensure the valve is sealed. Press the "Manual" button and cook at High Pressure for 3 minutes.
6.	When the cooking is done, quick release the pressure and carefully remove the lid.
7.	Carefully remove the salmon from your Instant Pot and transfer to serving plates.
8.	Serve and enjoy!
Nutrition information per serving:
- Calories: 254
- Fat: 8.8g
- Carbohydrates: 17.4g
- Protein: 27.5g
- Dietary Fiber: 0g

Flavorful Cod Fillets Taco Bowl

Time: 15 minutes
Servings: 3
Ingredients:
3 (5-ounce) cod fillets
1/2 cup of fresh green cabbage, finely shredded
1/4 cup of fresh red cabbage, finely shredded
2 medium carrots, peeled and grated
Freshly squeezed juice from 1 medium-sized lime
1/4 cup of fresh cilantro, finely chopped
2 tablespoons of fresh orange juice
1/2 teaspoon of garlic powder
1/2 teaspoon of sea salt
1 teaspoon of organic ground cumin
1 tablespoon of coconut oil
1 medium-sized ripe avocado, peeled and finely chopped
2 medium-sized zucchinis, finely chopped
1 cup of water
Instructions:
1.   Add 1 cup of water and a trivet to your Instant Pot.
2.   Season the cod fillets with sea salt and garlic powder. Place the cod fillets on top of the trivet.
3.   Lock the lid and ensure the valve is sealed. Press the "Manual" button and cook for 3 minutes at High Pressure.
4.   When the cooking is done, quick release the pressure and carefully remove the lid. Remove the cod from your Instant Pot.
5.   In a large bowl, add the rest of the ingredients and gently stir until fully combined.
6.   Distribute the slaw among 3 serving bowls and top with cod fillets.
7.   Serve and enjoy!
Nutrition information per serving:
- Calories: 485
- Fat: 36.5g
- Carbohydrates: 21.3g
- Protein: 24.8g
- Dietary Fiber: 12g

Elegant Curried Coconut Fish

Time: 26 minutes
Servings: 4
Ingredients:
1-1/2 pounds of boneless salmon or tilapia fish fillets, cut into small or large chunks
1 medium-sized zucchini, finely chopped
2 medium-sized red onions, sliced
3 garlic cloves, finely minced
1 tablespoon of fresh ginger, peeled and finely minced
1 teaspoon of organic ground cumin
1/2 teaspoon of organic turmeric
1 teaspoon of sea salt
Freshly squeezed juice from ½ medium-sized lemon
2 cups of unsweetened coconut milk
2 tablespoons of coconut oil
Instructions:
1.   Press the "Sauté" function on your Instant Pot and add the coconut oil.
2.   Once the oil is hot and ready, add the chopped red onion, minced garlic, and minced ginger. Sauté until softened, stirring occasionally.
3.   Add the seasoning and cook for another 2 minutes.
4.   Add the remaining ingredients to your Instant Pot and gently stir until combined.
5.   Lock the lid and ensure the valve is sealed. Press the "Manual" button and cook at Low for 5 minutes.
6.   When the cooking is done, naturally release the pressure and carefully remove the lid. Give the curry a good stir before serving.
7.   Serve and enjoy!
Nutrition information per serving:
- Calories: 594
- Fat: 46.1g
- Carbohydrates: 14.4g
- Protein: 37.1g
- Dietary Fiber: 4.6g

<u>Vegan and Vegetarian Recipes</u>

Journey Mashed Garlic Cauliflower

Time: 30 minutes
Servings: 6
Ingredients:
2 large cauliflower, roughly chopped
6 to 8 garlic cloves, finely minced
3/4 cup of unsweetened coconut cream or unsweetened coconut milk
2 cups of homemade low-sodium vegetable broth
2 tablespoons of ghee or coconut butter
1 teaspoon of sea salt
Instructions:
1.   Add a trivet and vegetable broth to your Instant Pot.
2.   Place the cauliflower on top of the trivet.
3.   Lock the lid and ensure the valve is sealed. Press the "Manual" button and cook at High Pressure for 3 minutes.
4.   When the cooking is done, quick release the pressure and carefully remove the lid.
5.   In a food processor, add the cauliflower, garlic, coconut cream, ghee, and sea salt. Pulse until smooth.
6.   Serve and enjoy!
Nutrition information per serving:
- Calories: 194
- Fat: 12.35g
- Carbohydrates: 5.96g
- Protein: 12.3g
- Dietary Fiber: 0g

World-Famous Cranberry Maple Brussel Sprouts

Time: 10 minutes
Servings: 4
Ingredients:
1-1/2 pounds of brussel sprouts, trimmed
2 cups of water
1 cup of fresh cranberries
3 tablespoons of pure maple syrup
3 tablespoons of coconut oil
2 tablespoons of dried rosemary
1 teaspoon of sea salt
Instructions:
1.   Add 2 cups of water and a steamer basket to your Instant Pot.
2.   In a large bowl, add the brussel sprouts, cranberries, pure maple syrup, coconut oil, dried rosemary, and sea salt.
3.   Place the brussel sprouts and cranberries in your steamer basket.
4.   Lock the lid and ensure the valve is sealed. Press the "Manual" button and cook at High Pressure for 2 minutes.
5.   When your Instant Pot timer beeps, quick release the pressure and carefully remove the lid.
6.   Serve and enjoy!
Nutrition information per serving:
- Calories: 217
- Fat: 10.9g
- Carbohydrates: 29.3g
- Protein: 6.1g
- Dietary Fiber:7.4g

Exotic Mashed Sweet Potatoes with Cranberry-Orange Sauce

Time: 27 minutes

Servings: 16

Cranberry-Orange Sauce Ingredients:

1 cup of water

1-1/2 cup of fresh cranberries

1/2 teaspoon of organic ground cinnamon

2 tablespoons of freshly squeezed orange juice

Mashed Sweet Potato Ingredients:

10 cups of sweet potatoes, peeled and cut into 1-inch chunks

1/4 cup of coconut butter or ghee

1/2 teaspoon of sea salt

1 cup of water or homemade low-sodium vegetable broth

Instructions:

1. Add 1 cup of water and a steamer basket to your Instant Pot.
2. Place the sweet potato chunks in the steamer basket and sprinkle with sea salt.
3. Lock the lid and ensure the valve is sealed. Press the "Manual" button and cook at High Pressure for 8 minutes.
4. When the cooking is done, quick release the pressure and carefully remove the lid.
5. Transfer the sweet potatoes to a large bowl and discard the steamer basket and liquid from your Instant Pot.
6. Use a potato masher to mash the sweet potatoes and gently stir in the coconut butter or ghee. Continue to mash the sweet potatoes until smooth.
7. Press the "Sauté" function on your Instant Pot and add the all the cranberry-orange sauce ingredients. Bring to a boil and reduce the temperature to low. Allow simmering until well heated through.
8. Drizzle the cranberry sauce over the sweet potatoes.
9. Serve and enjoy!

Nutrition information per serving:

- Calories: 147
- Fat: 3.6g
- Carbohydrates: 27.3g
- Protein: 1.4g
- Dietary Fiber: 4.2g

Globally-Known Spinach and Artichoke Dip

Time: 15 minutes
Servings: 2 cups
Ingredients:
1 (14-ounce) can of artichoke hearts, drained
2 zucchini squash, peeled and cut into 1/2-inch pieces
6 whole garlic cloves, peeled
1 large onion, roughly chopped
2 cups of spinach, roughly chopped
2 tablespoons of fresh dill, finely chopped
1 large lemon, juice
1 teaspoon of sea salt
1/4 cup of nutritional yeast
Instructions:
1.   Add the artichoke hearts, zucchini squash, garlic, onion, spinach, and sea salt to your Instant Pot.
2.   Lock the lid and ensure the valve is closed. Press the "Manual" button and cook at High Pressure for 4 minutes.
3.   When the cooking is done, quick release the pressure and carefully remove the lid.
4.   Transfer the contents to a blender along with the lemon juice and nutritional yeast. Pulse until smooth or reached your desired consistency.
Nutrition information per serving:
- Calories: 139
- Fat: 0.9g
- Carbohydrates: 30.3g
- Protein: 10.3g
- Dietary Fiber: 14g

Ambitious Steamed Vegetables

Time: 10 minutes
Servings: 6
Ingredients:
1 pound of carrots, peeled and thickly sliced
1 pound of brussel sprouts, trimmed and halved
1/2 pound of broccoli florets
1/2 pound of cauliflower florets
1/2 teaspoon of garlic powder
1/2 teaspoon of onion powder
Freshly squeezed juice from 1/2 medium-sized lemon
1 tablespoon of coconut oil
1 tablespoon of fresh parsley, finely chopped
1 teaspoon of sea salt
1 cup of water
Instructions:
1.   Add 1 cup of water and a steamer basket to your Instant Pot.
2.   Add the vegetables in the steamer basket and sprinkle the garlic powder, onion powder, and sea salt. Drizzle with lemon juice and coconut oil.
3.   Lock the lid and ensure the valve is closed. Press the "Manual" button and cook at High Pressure for 2 minutes.
4.   When the cooking is done, naturally release the pressure for 5 minutes before quick releasing the rest of the pressure.
5.   Transfer the vegetables to a large bowl and sprinkle with fresh parsley. Give a good stir.
6.   Serve and enjoy!
Nutrition information per serving:
- Calories: 95
- Fat: 3.63g
- Carbohydrates: 15.3g
- Protein: 4.3g
- Dietary Fiber: 4.8g

Wonderful Sri Lankan Coconut Cabbage

Time: 30 minutes
Servings: 4
Ingredients:
1 tablespoon of coconut oil or avocado oil
3 garlic cloves, minced
1 medium-sized yellow or sweet onion, thinly sliced
1 teaspoon of sea salt
1 medium-sized green cabbage, cored and finely shredded
2 tablespoons of freshly squeezed lemon juice
1/2 cup of unsweetened desiccated coconut
1 tablespoon of organic turmeric powder
1/3 cup of homemade low-sodium vegetable broth
Instructions:
1.   Press the "Sauté" function on your Instant Pot and add the coconut oil.
2.   Add the onion and sauté for 4 minutes or until softened, stirring occasionally.
3.   Add the garlic and sauté for 30 seconds, stirring occasionally.
4.   Add the remaining ingredients to your Instant Pot.
5.   Lock the lid and ensure the valve is closed. Press the "Manual" button and cook at High Pressure for 5 minutes.
6.   When the cooking is done, naturally release the pressure for 5 minutes before quick releasing the rest of the pressure. Carefully remove the lid.
7.   Serve and enjoy!
Nutrition information per serving:
*   Calories: 157
*   Fat: 7.1g
*   Carbohydrates: 22.9g
*   Protein: 4.8g
*   Dietary Fiber: 9.3g

The Best Garlic "Butter" Mushrooms

Time: 20 minutes
Servings: 4
Ingredients:
2 pounds of button mushrooms
2 tablespoon of coconut oil
4 tablespoons of coconut butter or ghee
4 garlic cloves, minced
1 tablespoon of fresh thyme, finely chopped
1 tablespoon of fresh parsley, finely chopped
1/2 teaspoon of sea salt
Instructions:
1.   Press the "Sauté" function on your Instant Pot and add the coconut oil.
2.   Once the oil is hot, add the mushrooms and sauté for 5 minutes, stirring occasionally.
3.   Add the minced garlic, coconut butter, fresh thyme, fresh parsley, and sea salt. Mix until well coated together.
4.   Lock the lid and ensure the valve is closed. Press the "Manual" button and cook at High Pressure for 13 minutes.
5.   When the cooking is done, naturally release the pressure for 5 minutes before quick releasing the rest of the pressure. Carefully remove the lid.
6.   Transfer the mushrooms to a serving platter and ladle the butter sauce over.
7.   Serve and enjoy!
Nutrition information per serving:
*   Calories: 195
*   Fat: 16.8g
*   Carbohydrates: 8.4g
*   Protein: 7.4g
*   Dietary Fiber: 2.3g

Mulligatawny

Time: 30 minutes
Servings: 6

Ingredients:
2 tablespoons of coconut oil or avocado oil
1 red onion, finely chopped
4 garlic cloves, minced
1 tablespoon of fresh ginger, minced
1 medium-sized cauliflower, roughly chopped
2 medium-sized apples, peeled, cored, and chopped
1 large sweet potato, cut into 1-inch pieces
1/2 green cabbage, cored and finely chopped
4 cups of homemade low-sodium vegetable broth
1 cup of unsweetened coconut milk
1 teaspoon of sea salt
1 medium-sized lime, juice

Blender Ingredients:
1/2 teaspoon of fenugreek
1 teaspoon of organic cinnamon
3 whole garlic cloves
1 tablespoon of turmeric
1 tablespoon of fresh ginger, peeled and minced
2 tablespoons of fresh cilantro, minced

Instructions:
1. Press the "Sauté" function on your Instant Pot and add the coconut oil.
2. In a blender, add all the blender ingredients and blend until smooth.
3. When the oil is hot and ready, add the chopped red onion, minced garlic, minced ginger, and ½ of the curry seasoning. Sauté for 6 minutes or until softened, stirring occasionally.
4. Add cauliflower, apple, sweet potato, cabbage, vegetable broth, coconut milk, sea salt, lime juice, and remaining curry powder seasoning.
5. Lock the lid and ensure the valve is sealed. Press the "Manual" button and cook at High Pressure for 8 minutes.
6. When the cooking is done, allow for a full natural release and carefully remove the lid. Gently stir until everything is combined.
7. Serve and enjoy!

Nutrition information per serving:
- Calories: 244
- Fat: 14.6g
- Carbohydrates: 28.9g
- Protein: 4.8g
- Dietary Fiber: 8.1g

Peaceful Green Curry

Time: 11 minutes

Servings: 4

Ingredients:

3 medium-sized sweet potatoes, cut into bite-sized pieces

1 cup of broccoli florets

1 cup of cauliflower florets

1 cup of spinach

2 cups of homemade low-sodium vegetable broth

1/2 cup of frozen peas

1 teaspoon of garlic powder

1 teaspoon of onion powder

2 tablespoons of green curry paste

1 cup of unsweetened coconut milk

1 teaspoon of sea salt

Instructions:

1.   Add the sweet potatoes, broccoli, cauliflower, and 1 cup of vegetable broth to your Instant Pot.

2.   Lock the lid and ensure the valve is sealed. Press the "Manual" button and cook at High Pressure for 3 minutes.

3.   When the cooking is done, quick release the pressure and carefully remove the lid.

4.   Press the "Sauté" function on your Instant Pot and add the remaining ingredients. Gently stir until combined.

5.   Allow cooking until the curry is heated through and the spinach has wilted through.

6.   Serve and enjoy!

Nutrition information per serving:

- Calories: 324
- Fat: 16.2g
- Carbohydrates: 42.7g
- Protein: 5.4g
- Dietary Fiber: 8.2g

Courageous Kung Pao Cauliflower

Time: 25 minutes
Servings: 4
Ingredients:
2 tablespoons of coconut oil or avocado oil
1 large head of cauliflower, cut into florets
3 medium-sized zucchinis, spiralized
1 large carrot, peeled and julienned
1 tablespoon of fresh ginger, peeled and minced
2 garlic cloves, minced
6 scallions, cut into 2-inch pieces
1 teaspoon of sea salt
2 tablespoons of white wine vinegar
2 tablespoons of organic pureed pumpkin
4 tablespoons of low-sodium coconut aminos
2 tablespoons of raw honey
3 teaspoons of coconut flour
1/4 cup of homemade low-sodium vegetable broth or water
Instructions:
1.   In a bowl, add the white wine vinegar, pureed pumpkin, coconut aminos, raw honey, coconut flour, and vegetable broth or water. Mix well and set aside.
2.   Press the "Sauté" function on your Instant Pot and add the coconut oil.
3.   Once the oil is hot, add the cauliflower and cook for 5 minutes, stirring occasionally.
4.   Remove the cauliflower and set aside.
5.   Add the julienned carrots to your Instant Pot and sauté for 3 minutes, stirring occasionally.
6.   Return the cauliflower to your Instant Pot along with the ginger and garlic. Sauté for another 2 minutes.
7.   Turn off the "Sauté" function on your Instant Pot. The Instant Pot will still be hot so add the spiralized zucchini, sauce, sea salt, and scallions. Saute until the zucchini noodles are well heated through. Do not overcook as it will result in a mushy texture.
8.   Serve and enjoy!
Nutrition information per serving:
*   Calories: 333
*   Fat: 13.5g
*   Carbohydrates: 48.3g
*   Protein: 5g
*   Dietary Fiber: 6.39g

Relaxed Mushroom and Asparagus Stir-Fry

Time: 9 minutes
Servings: 4
Ingredients:
1 pound of asparagus, cut into 1 to 2-inch pieces
1 pound of mushrooms, quartered
2 tablespoons of coconut oil
Sauce Ingredients:
1/2 cup of homemade low-sodium vegetable broth
2 tablespoons of low-sodium coconut aminos
2 garlic cloves, minced
Instructions:
1.   In a small bowl, add the vegetable broth, coconut aminos, and garlic. Mix well.
2.   Press the "Sauté" function on your Instant Pot and add the coconut oil.
3.   Once the oil is hot, add the mushrooms and cook for 2 minutes, stirring occasionally.
4.   Add the asparagus and cook for an extra 4 minutes, stirring occasionally.
5.   Add the sauce and continue to cook until the sauce is heated through with the vegetables.
6.   Turn off the "Sauté" Setting and transfer the vegetables to a serving plate.
7.   Serve and enjoy!
Nutrition information per serving:
- Calories: 107
- Fat: 7.6g
- Carbohydrates: 8.3g
- Protein: 6.1g
- Dietary Fiber: 3.1g

Lively Ginger-Flavored Cabbage and Carrots

Time: 15 minutes
Servings: 6
Ingredients:
1 medium-sized head of green cabbage, cored and finely shredded
2 tablespoons of coconut oil or avocado oil
4 garlic cloves, minced
2 cups of carrots, julienned
1 tablespoon of fresh ginger, peeled and minced
1 tablespoon of apple cider vinegar
1 tablespoon of low-sodium coconut aminos
1 cup of homemade low-sodium vegetable broth
1 teaspoon of sea salt
Instructions:
1.   Press the "Sauté" function on your Instant Pot and add the coconut oil.
2.   Once the oil is hot, add the ginger and garlic. Cook for 1 minute or until fragrant, stirring occasionally.
3.   Turn off the "Sauté" function on your Instant Pot and add the remaining ingredients.
4.   Lock the lid and ensure the valve is closed. Press the "Manual" button and cook for 7 minutes at High Pressure.
5.   When the cooking is done, quick release the pressure and carefully remove the lid.
6.   Serve and enjoy!
Nutrition information per serving:
- Calories: 93
- Fat: 3g
- Carbohydrates: 21.2g
- Protein: 5.63g
- Dietary Fiber: 2.32g

Pleasant Vegan AIP-Friendly Carrot and Sweet Potato Chili

Time: 25 minutes

Servings: 6

Ingredients:

4 cups of sweet potatoes, cut into bite-sized pieces

4 cups of homemade low-sodium beef broth, chicken broth, or vegetable broth

2 cups of carrots, cut into 1 to 2-inch pieces

8 garlic cloves, minced

1 medium-sized onion, finely chopped

2 tablespoons of olive oil or coconut oil

1 tablespoon of fresh thyme

1 teaspoon of sea salt

1 teaspoon of freshly cracked black pepper

Instructions:

1. Press the "Sauté" function on your Instant Pot and add the olive oil.
2. Once the oil is hot and ready, add the onions and sauté until translucent.
3. Add the garlic to your Instant Pot and cook for an additional minute.
4. Add the ground beef and cook until almost brown.
5. Add the sweet potatoes and carrots and cook for another 3 to 5 minutes.
6. Add the remaining ingredients and give a gentle stir.
7. Lock the lid and ensure the valve is closed. Press the "Manual" button and cook for 8 minutes at High Pressure.
8. When the cooking is done, allow for a 5-minute natural release before quick releasing the remaining pressure.
9. If you prefer, use the "Sauté" function on your Instant Pot to simmer the chili until reached your desired consistency. Adjust the seasoning if necessary.
10. Serve and enjoy!

Nutrition information per serving:

- Calories: 212
- Fat: 5.8g
- Carbohydrates: 35.1g
- Protein: 5.5g
- Dietary Fiber: 5.5g

Perfectly Prepared Apple and Pork Meatloaf

Time: 1 hour
Servings: 6
Ingredients:
1-1/2 pounds of ground pork
1 medium-sized apple, peeled and chopped
6 medium-sized slices of bacon
3/4 cup of unsweetened homemade applesauce
2 to 4 tablespoons of coconut flour
1 small red onion, finely chopped
1 teaspoon of organic ground cinnamon powder
1 teaspoon of sea salt
1 cup of water or homemade low-sodium beef broth
Instructions:
1.   In a large bowl, add the ground pork, apple, unsweetened applesauce, coconut flour, onion, cinnamon, and sea salt. Mix until well combined.
2.   Form the ground pork mixture into a loaf.
3.   Arrange the bacon on top of the loaf.
4.   Add 1 cup of water and a trivet to your Instant Pot.
5.   Place the meatloaf on the trivet.
6.   Lock the lid and ensure the valve is closed. Press the "Manual" button and cook at High Pressure for 40 minutes.
7.   When the cooking is done, allow for a full natural release before removing the lid.
8.   Transfer the meatloaf to a baking sheet.
9.   Broil inside a broiler for 3 to 5 minutes or until brown and crispy on top.
10.   Serve and enjoy!
Nutrition information per serving:
- Calories: 345
- Fat: 13g
- Carbohydrates: 17.2g
- Protein: 38.4g
- Dietary Fiber: 5.7g

Optimum Sautéed Radishes with Garlic

Time: 20 minutes
Servings: 4
Ingredients:
1 pound of radishes, trimmed and quartered
2 tablespoons of coconut oil
1 tablespoon of fresh parsley, finely chopped
4 to 6 garlic cloves, minced
1 teaspoon of sea salt
Instructions:
1.   Select the "Sauté" setting on your Instant Pot and add the coconut oil.
2.   When the oil is hot, add the radishes and garlic. Sauté for 10 to 15 minutes or until the radishes are tender, stirring occasionally.
3.   Sprinkle fresh parsley and sea salt.
4.   Serve and enjoy!
Nutrition information per serving:
- Calories: 84
- Fat: 6.9g
- Carbohydrates: 5.4g
- Protein: 1.1g
- Dietary Fiber: 1.9g

Ideal Cinnamon-Honey Carrots

Time: 10 minutes
Servings: 8

2 pounds of baby carrots
1/2 cup of homemade low-sodium vegetable broth
2 tablespoons of coconut oil
1-1/2 teaspoon of organic ground cinnamon powder
1/4 cup of raw honey
1/2 teaspoon of pure vanilla extract
1 teaspoon of sea salt

Instructions:

1. Add the baby carrots to your Instant Pot with the vegetable broth. Sprinkle with sea salt.
2. Lock the lid and ensure the valve is sealed. Press the "Manual" button and cook at High Pressure for 2 minutes.
3. When your Instant Pot timer beeps, quick release the pressure. Carefully remove the lid.
4. Drain the broth from your Instant Pot and return to your Instant Pot.
5. In a small bowl, add and combine the coconut oil, cinnamon, honey, and vanilla extract.
6. Pour the mixture over the carrots and gently stir until fully coated with the honey mixture.
7. Serve and enjoy!

Nutrition information per serving:

- Calories: 101
- Fat: 3.6g
- Carbohydrates: 18.1g
- Protein: 0.8g
- Dietary Fiber: 3.3g

Side Dishes and Desserts Recipes

Generous Coconut Yogurt

Time: 15 minutes plus refrigerating time.
Servings: 6
Ingredients:
2 cans of unsweetened coconut cream
2 teaspoons of gelatin
2 (pint-sized) ball jars, sterilized
Instructions:
1.   Add the coconut cream to the heatproof jars.
2.   Add the jars to your Instant Pot.
3.   Cover and seal the lid. Select the "Yogurt" setting and set the time to 12 minutes. Press start.
4.   When the timer beeps, carefully remove the lid and remove the yogurt.
5.   Add the yogurt to a blender along with the gelatin. Blend until combined and return to the jars.
6.   Add the jars to your refrigerator and allow to cool until thickened.
7.   Serve and enjoy!
Nutrition information per serving:
- Calories: 367
- Fat: 38.1g
- Carbohydrates: 8.9g
- Protein: 3.5g
- Dietary Fiber: 5.6g

Traditional Cauliflower Cinnamon Oatmeal

Time: 5 minutes
Servings: 4
Ingredients:
4 cups of cauliflower rice
2 cups of unsweetened coconut milk
2 tablespoons of coconut flour
2 teaspoons of organic ground cinnamon powder
1/2 teaspoon of nutmeg
1/4 cup of pure maple syrup
Instructions:
1.   Add all the ingredients except for coconut flour to your Instant Pot and gently stir until fully combined.
2.   Cover and seal the lid. Press the "Manual" button and cook for 2 minutes at High Pressure.
3.   When the cooking is done, quick release the pressure and remove the lid.
4.   Sprinkle 2 tablespoons of coconut flour and gently stir until thickens.
5.   Transfer to bowls.
6.   Serve and enjoy!
Nutrition information per serving:
- Calories: 310
- Fat: 20g
- Carbohydrates: 30g
- Protein: 9g
- Dietary Fiber: 5g

Modern Raspberry Chocolate Chip Mug Cakes

Time: 10 minutes
Servings: 2
Ingredients:
1/3 cup of coconut flour
1 tablespoon of coconut oil
3 tablespoons of unsweetened coconut milk
1 teaspoon of baking powder
2 tablespoons of unsweetened chocolate chips
1/2 cup of frozen or fresh raspberries
A small pinch of sea salt
Instructions:
1.   Add all the ingredients to a large bowl and gently stir until fully combined.
2.   Grease a heatproof jar or ramekin with nonstick cooking spray.
3.   Divide the batter and add to the ramekin.
4.   Add 1 cup of water and a trivet to your Instant Pot.
5.   Place the ramekins on top and cover with aluminum foil.
6.   Close and seal the lid. Press the "Manual" button and cook for 10 minutes at High Pressure.
7.   When the cooking is done, quick release the pressure and remove the lid.
8.   Serve and enjoy!
Nutrition information per serving:
- Calories: 423
- Fat: 21.6g
- Carbohydrates: 51.2g
- Protein: 9.7g
- Dietary Fiber: 27.9g

Wicked Pumpkin Custard

Time: 15 minutes
Servings: 2
Ingredients:
2 cups of organic pureed pumpkins
1-3/4 cups of unsweetened coconut milk
1 teaspoon of pumpkin pie spice
1 teaspoon of organic ground cinnamon powder
1/2-inch of fresh ginger, peeled and finely minced
1 teaspoon of organic vanilla extract
1/4 teaspoon of sea salt
Instructions:
1.   In a medium bowl, add the pureed pumpkins, coconut milk, pumpkin pie spice, cinnamon powder, minced ginger, vanilla extract, and sea salt. Gently stir until fully combined.
2.   Add the mixture to a greased heatproof bowl.
3.   Add 1 cup of water and a trivet to your Instant Pot.
4.   Tightly cover the heatproof bowl with aluminum foil and place on the trivet.
5.   Close and seal the lid. Press the "Manual" button and cook for 7 minutes at High Pressure.
6.   When your Instant Pot beeps, naturally release the pressure for 10 minutes before manually releasing the rest of the pressure.
7.   Serve and enjoy!
Nutrition information per serving:
- Calories: 577
- Fat: 50.8g
- Carbohydrates: 31.6g
- Protein: 7.6g
- Dietary Fiber: 11.7g

Terrific Bacon Jam

Time: 30 minutes
Servings: 16
Ingredients:
1 pound of bacon, finely chopped
1 large yellow onion, finely chopped
4 garlic cloves, halved
1/4 cup of apple cider vinegar
1/2 cup of organic honey or pure maple syrup
1/2 cup of water
Instructions:
1.   Press the "Sauté" setting on your Instant Pot and add the bacon and onions. Cook until onions are translucent and bacon has browned, stirring occasionally.
2.   Add the garlic and cook for 1 more minute.
3.   Turn off the "Sauté" function and discard the bacon grease.
4.   Add the remaining ingredients to your Instant Pot and gently stir until fully combined.
5.   Lock the lid and press the "Manual" button. Cook at high pressure for 10 minutes.
6.   When the cooking is done, manually release the pressure and remove the lid.
7.   Use an immersion blender to blend the contents until smooth or reached your desired consistency.
8.   Spoon the bacon jam to a mason jar and refrigerate.
9.   Serve and enjoy!
Nutrition information per serving:
- Calories: 189
- Fat: 11.9g
- Carbohydrates: 9.8g
- Protein: 10.7g
- Dietary Fiber: 0.2g

Appreciative Carrot Pudding

Time: 15 minutes
Servings: 4
Ingredients:
4 cups of grated carrots
1/2 cup of unsweetened coconut milk
1/4 cup of water
4 tablespoons of ghee or coconut oil
1/2 teaspoon of organic honey or pure maple syrup
1/2 teaspoon of organic ground cinnamon powder
Instructions:
1.   Add all the ingredients except for the ghee to your Instant Pot and gently stir until fully combined.
2.   Close and seal the lid. Press the "Manual" button and cook for 1 minute at High Pressure.
3.   When the cooking is done, manually release the pressure and remove the lid.
4.   Press the "Sauté" function on your Instant Pot and cook for 6 minutes or until the liquid evaporated.
5.   Stir in the ghee and sauté for an additional 6 to 8 minutes.
6.   Serve and enjoy!
Nutrition information per serving:
- Calories: 231
- Fat: 20.8g
- Carbohydrates: 12.6g
- Protein: 1.6g
- Dietary Fiber: 3.4g

Proud Apricot Crisp

Time: 15 minutes
Servings: 4
Ingredients:
3 cups of apricots, pitted and chopped
2 tablespoons of pure raw honey or maple syrup
Crumb Topping Ingredients:
1/4 cup of coconut butter
1/3 cup of coconut flour
A small pinch of sea salt
Instructions:
1. Add the apricots and honey to the bottom of your Instant Pot.
2. In a medium bowl, add and mix the coconut butter, coconut flour, and sea salt. Set aside.
3. Lock the lid on your Instant Pot and press the "Manual" button and cook for 3 minutes at High Pressure.
4. When the cooking is done, manually release the pressure and carefully remove the lid.
5. Transfer the apricots to a pan and spread the crumble topping.
6. Broil until golden brown and crisp on top.
7. Serve and enjoy!

Nutrition information per serving:
- Calories: 348
- Fat: 20.7g
- Carbohydrates: 40.9g
- Protein: 9g
- Dietary Fiber: 14.8g

Fantastic Caramel Sauce

Time: 22 minutes
Servings: About 2 cups
Ingredients:
1/4 cup of coconut oil
1 (14-ounce) can of unsweetened coconut cream
3/4 cup of pure maple syrup
1 teaspoon of vanilla extract
1/8 teaspoon of sea salt
Instructions:
1. Select the "Sauté" function on your Instant Pot and add all the ingredients.
2. Stir until smooth and bring to a boil.
3. Boil inside your Instant Pot for 15 minutes, stirring occasionally.
4. Turn off the "Sauté" function on your Instant Pot.
5. Cool slightly and spoon into mason jars.
6. Serve and enjoy!

Nutrition information per serving:
- Calories: 931
- Fat: 74.8g
- Carbohydrates: 90.2g
- Protein: 4.6g
- Dietary Fiber: 4.4g

Innovative Ginger Applesauce

Time: 5 minutes
Servings: 12
Ingredients:
12 medium-sized apples, chopped
3/4 cup of water
2 tablespoons of fresh ginger, peeled and minced
1 tablespoon of organic ground cinnamon powder
1 tablespoon of organic honey or pure maple syrup
Freshly squeezed juice of a ½ medium-sized lemon
2 tablespoons of ghee
1/4 teaspoon of sea salt
Instructions:
1.   Add all the ingredients to your Instant Pot.
2.   Cover and seal the lid. Press the "Manual" button and cook for 3 minutes at High Pressure.
3.   When the cooking is done, naturally release the pressure and remove the lid.
4.   Use an immersion blender to blend the applesauce until smooth or reached your desired consistency.
5.   Refrigerate until cool.
6.   Serve and enjoy!
Nutrition information per serving:
- Calories: 116
- Fat: 0.4g
- Carbohydrates: 30.8g
- Protein: 0.7g
- Dietary Fiber: 5.4g

Captivating Berry Compote

Time: 5 minutes
Servings: 4
Ingredients:
1 pound of fresh strawberries, trimmed and halved
1 pound of fresh blueberries
2 teaspoons of fresh lemon juice
2 teaspoons of fresh orange juice
Instructions:
1.   Add all the ingredients to your Instant Pot.
2.   Cover and seal the lid. Press the "Manual" button and cook for 1 minute at High Pressure.
3.   When the cooking is done, allow for a full natural release and carefully remove the lid.
4.   Allow the berry compote to thicken.
5.   If you prefer, refrigerate until cool.
6.   Serve and enjoy!
Nutrition information per serving:
- Calories: 101
- Fat: 0.7g
- Carbohydrates: 25.1g
- Protein: 1.7g
- Dietary Fiber: 5g

Dressings, Sauces and Condiments Recipes

Presenting Beet Dip

Time: 55 minutes
Servings: 16
Ingredients:
2 pounds of beets, peeled and cut into 1-inch pieces
1 cup of low-sodium vegetable broth or water
1 tablespoon of apple cider vinegar
1/4 cup of fresh lemon juice
2 garlic cloves
1/3 cup of olive oil
1 tablespoon of coconut oil or coconut butter
1/2 teaspoon of sea salt
Instructions:
1.   Add the beets, vegetable broth, apple cider vinegar, lemon juice, garlic cloves, coconut oil, and sea salt to your Instant Pot.
2.   Cover and seal the lid. Press the "Manual" button and cook for 40 minutes at High Pressure.
3.   When the cooking is done, quick release or naturally release the pressure. Remove the lid.
4.   Gently stir everything together.
5.   Strain the beet mixture over a large bowl and reserve the broth.
6.   In a food processor or blender, add the beet mixture with the olive oil and broth. Process until smooth or reached your desired consistency.
7.   Serve and enjoy!
Nutrition information per serving:
- Calories: 73
- Fat: 5.3g
- Carbohydrates: 5.9g
- Protein: 1.3g
- Dietary Fiber: 1.2g

Honorable Sausage Gravy

Time: 15 minutes
Servings: 6
Ingredients:
1 pound of ground sausage
2 medium-sized bacon slices, finely chopped
1/2 cup of homemade low-sodium chicken broth or chicken stock
1/2 cup of coconut flour
3 cups of unsweetened coconut milk
1/2 teaspoon of sea salt
1/2 teaspoon of freshly cracked black pepper
Instructions:
1. Press the "Sauté" function on your Instant Pot.
2. Once hot, add the ground sausage and bacon to your Instant Pot. Cook until brown, typically around 5 minutes.
3. Gently stir in the chicken broth.
4. Cover and seal the lid. Press the "Manual" button and cook for 5 minutes at High Pressure.
5. When the cooking is done, naturally release or quick release the pressure. Remove the lid.
6. In a medium bowl, mix together the coconut flour and coconut milk.
7. Press the "Sauté" function on your Instant Pot and pour in the milk mixture.
8. Season with sea salt and freshly cracked black pepper.
9. Gently stir until the gravy is thick. Turn off your Instant Pot.
10. Serve and enjoy!
Nutrition information per serving:
- Calories: 610
- Fat: 53.8g
- Carbohydrates: 13.5g
- Protein: 6.6g
- Dietary Fiber: 21.5g

Definitive Cauliflower Gravy

Time: 10 minutes
Servings: 4
Ingredients:
1 large cauliflower head, cut into florets
1 cups of homemade low-sodium chicken broth
1 cup of unsweetened coconut milk
2 tablespoons of coconut flour (optional)
2 garlic cloves, minced
1 teaspoon of sea salt
1 teaspoon of crushed dried rosemary
Instructions:
1. Add the cauliflower florets, chicken broth, coconut milk, minced garlic, salt, and dried rosemary to your Instant Pot.
2. Cover and seal the lid. Press the "Manual" button and cook for 10 minutes at High Pressure.
3. When the cooking is done, naturally release the pressure and remove the lid.
4. Use an immersion blender to blend the cauliflower until smooth.You can sprinkle the coconut flour for a thicker gravy.
5. Season with salt and black pepper.
6. Serve and enjoy!
Nutrition information per serving:
- Calories: 150
- Fat: 14.9g
- Carbohydrates: 15.2g
- Protein: 6.6g
- Dietary Fiber: 6.8g

Universally Loved Barbeque Sauce

Time: 10 minutes
Servings: 4
Ingredients:
1 cup of pureed pumpkin or unsweetened applesauce
1 tablespoon of balsamic vinegar
1 tablespoon of extra-virgin olive oil or coconut oil
1 tablespoon of molasses
1/3 cup of pure maple syrup
3 garlic cloves, crushed
3 tablespoons of apple cider vinegar
1 tablespoon of low-sodium coconut aminos
1 teaspoon of fresh ginger, finely minced
1 teaspoon of sea salt
Instructions:
1.   Press the "Sauté" function on your Instant Pot and add the oil.
2.   Once hot, add the minced garlic and minced ginger. Sauté until fragrant, stirring occasionally.
3.   Turn off the "Sauté" function on your Instant Pot.
4.   Gently stir in the remaining ingredients. Cover and seal the lid. Press the "Manual" button and cook for 6 minutes at High Pressure.
5.   When the cooking is done, allow for a full natural release and remove the lid.
6.   Store the barbeque sauce in a glass jar or container.
7.   Serve and enjoy!
Nutrition information per serving:
- Calories: 135
- Fat: 3.7g
- Carbohydrates: 26.3g
- Protein: 1.8g
- Dietary Fiber: 0.7g

Wild Cherry Barbecue Sauce

Time: 40 minutes
Servings: 3 cups
Ingredients:
2 tablespoons of olive oil or coconut oil
1 large yellow onion or sweet onion, roughly chopped
6 whole medium-sized garlic cloves, minced
3 cups of fresh or frozen cherries, pitted and halved
1/4 cup of pure raw honey or organic maple syrup
1/4 cup of organic apple cider vinegar
1 teaspoon of sea salt
Instructions:
1.   Press the "Sauté" function on your Instant Pot and add the olive oil or coconut oil.
2.   Once the oil is hot and ready, add the onion and sauté until browned, typically around 6 to 8 minutes.
3.   Add the garlic and sauté for 1 minute or until fragrant, stirring occasionally.
4.   Add the halved cherries, syrup, apple cider vinegar, and sea salt.
5.   Cover and seal the lid. Press the "Manual" button and cook for 5 minutes at High Pressure.
6.   When the cooking is done, naturally release the pressure and remove the lid.
7.   Transfer the contents to a blender and blend until smooth or fully combined.
8.   Store in jars or containers.
Nutrition information per serving:
- Calories: 422
- Fat: 9.6g
- Carbohydrates: 84.4g
- Protein: 2.2g
- Dietary Fiber: 1.7g

<u>Chapter 4: Autoimmune Protocol (AIP) Diet 3-Week Meal Plan</u>

In this chapter, you will find an effective 3-week Autoimmune Protocol meal plan that will last you for 3-weeks. This meal plan will provide you with a wide variety of recipes for you to enjoy each day. You are welcome to change the meal plan according to your liking. Enjoy!

Week One

Day One
- Meal one: Optimum Chicken and Apple Meatballs
- Meal two: Five-Star Onion Soup
- Meal three: Luxurious White Chicken Chili

Day Two
- Meal one: Highly Regarded Cauliflower and Sweet Potato Breakfast Hash
- Meal two: Yummy Apple Ginger Butternut Squash Soup
- Meal three: To-Die-For Ground Beef Stroganoff

Day Three
- Meal one: Palatable Maple Bacon Banana Breakfast Muffins
- Meal two: Ideal Cinnamon-Honey Carrots
- Meal three: Marathon Chinese-Inspired Ginger Fish

Day Four
- Meal one: Morning Sweet Potato Breakfast Bowls
- Meal two: Insanely Delicious Sweet Potato Soup
- Meal three: Elegant Curried Coconut Fish

Day Five
- Meal one: Gratifying Kale Butternut Squash and Pancetta Breakfast Hash
- Meal two: Optimum Sautéed Radishes with Garlic
- Meal three: Soulfully Apple Shredded Chicken

Day Six
- Meal one: Generous Coconut Yogurt
- Meal two: Kind Tilapia Fish Packets
- Meal three: Mulligatawny

Day Seven
- Meal one: Perfectly Spiced Apple Cider
- Meal two: Ambitious Steamed Vegetables
- Meal three: Glorious Lemon Salmon

Week Two

Day One
- Meal one: Highly Regarded Cauliflower and Sweet Potato Breakfast Hash
- Meal two: Enjoyable Kale and Pork Salad
- Meal three: Confident Chicken with Apples, Carrots, and Plums

Day Two
- Meal one: Healthy Green Detox Smoothie
- Meal two: Courageous Kung Pao Cauliflower
- Meal three: Pleasant Vegan AIP-Friendly Carrot and Sweet Potato Chili

Day Three
- Meal one: Refreshing! Agua De Jamaica "Hibiscus Tea"
- Meal two: Ambitious Steamed Vegetables
- Meal three: Desirable Filipino-Inspired Adobo Chicken

Day Four
- Meal one: Energizing Apple Carrot Banana Smoothie
- Meal two: Flavorful Cod Fillets Taco Bowl
- Meal three: Fit for a King Creamy Ground Beef Sweet Potato Stew

Day Five
- Meal one: Sunrise Pineapple Smoothie
- Meal two: Fascinating Beet Salad with Arugula

- Meal three: <u>Important Mango Chicken</u>

Day Six
- Meal one: <u>Wonderful Sri Lankan Coconut Cabbage</u>
- Meal two: <u>Captivating Steamed Broccoli Salad with Apple</u>
- Meal three: <u>Rockstar Balsamic Apple Pork Chops</u>

Day Seven
- Meal one: <u>Traditional Cauliflower Cinnamon Oatmeal</u>
- Meal two: <u>Very Creamy Chicken Chowder with Bacon</u>
- Meal three: <u>Dreamy Beef Goulash</u>

Week Three

Day One
- Meal one: <u>Fascinating Beet Salad with Arugula</u>
- Meal two: <u>Fit for a King Creamy Ground Beef Sweet Potato Stew</u>
- Meal three: <u>Marathon Chinese-Inspired Ginger Fish</u>

Day Two
- Meal one: <u>Gratifying Kale Butternut Squash and Pancetta Breakfast Hash</u>
- Meal two: <u>Amazingly Tasty Turmeric Chicken</u>
- Meal three: <u>Immersive Cranberry Creamy Beef Chili</u>

Day Three
- Meal one: <u>Energizing Apple Carrot Banana Smoothie</u>
- Meal two: <u>Determined Carrot Salad with Dried Cranberries and Pineapples</u>
- Meal three: <u>Only the Greatest Ginger-Balsamic Chicken</u>

Day Four
- Meal one: <u>Delicious Blueberry Coconut Smoothie</u>
- Meal two: <u>Relaxed Mushroom and Asparagus Stir-Fry</u>
- Meal three: <u>Immersive Cranberry Creamy Beef Chili</u>

Day Five
- Meal one: <u>Everyday Avocado Coconut Smoothie</u>
- Meal two: <u>Thoughtful Sweet Potato Salad</u>
- Meal three: <u>Considerate Honey Garlic Chicken</u>

Day Six
- Meal one: <u>Comforting Coleslaw Salad with Pulled Chicken</u>
- Meal two: <u>Beautiful Carrot Soup with Lemongrass</u>
- Meal three: <u>Defining 40-Garlic Clove Chicken</u>

Day Seven
- Meal one: <u>Palatable Maple Bacon Banana Breakfast Muffins</u>
- Meal two: <u>Innovative Ginger Applesauce</u>
- Meal three: <u>Agreeable Roasted Lemon Beef</u>

Remember if you don't feel like preparing a specific recipe you are free to change this meal plan depending on your preference. When locating these delicious recipes, please refer to the Table of Contents at the beginning of the book or click on the link.